BIG BREATH IN

A MEMOIR

The Fight to Breathe
and the Journey to a
Double-Lung Transplant

GEORGE KEULEN

◆ FriesenPress

One Printers Way
Altona, MB R0G 0B0
Canada

www.friesenpress.com

Copyright © 2021 by George Keulen
First Edition — 2021

All rights reserved.

No part of this publication may be reproduced in any form, or by any means, electronic or mechanical, including photocopying, recording, or any information browsing, storage, or retrieval system, without permission in writing from FriesenPress.

ISBN
978-1-03-911147-9 (Hardcover)
978-1-03-911146-2 (Paperback)
978-1-03-911148-6 (eBook)

Biography & Autobiography, Medical

Distributed to the trade by The Ingram Book Company

*For Kim,
my beloved*

PREFACE

"I would not but, alas, I must."
(*The Dyer's Hand and Other Essays*, W.H. Auden)

WHY WRITE A book? This is a question I have been coming back to again and again for over a decade. From the time I became critically ill in 2009 and began writing a blog to keep family and friends updated on how I was doing, people have been telling me to write a book. But what kind of book could I possibly write? What would be my thesis, my message?

Growing up, I was never one for books. It was not until my recovery from a transplant that I became an avid reader. I have also never enjoyed writing. Anyone who receives emails from me, or any professor who has had to grade a paper of mine, will tell you that my sentence structure is horrible, my grammar worse, and without spellcheck, my writing would be impossible to read—even spellcheck can't figure out everything I type.

So why would someone like me write a book and think that their life is worth putting down on paper? Well, there are many reasons. For one, even before my transplant, I felt that my life story had some unique aspects to it that some people might find interesting. Second, over the years, I have felt something of a "call" to get my CF and transplant story down on paper. But the biggest motivating factor was that the chorus of people telling me to write about my life simply became too loud to ignore.

I understand why people have encouraged me to write. There is something about *story* that is fundamental to who we are as people. For the most part, we as human beings love stories. Stories help us make sense of life, help us relate to others, and in stories, we find inspiration, courage, and comfort for our own experiences. At a time in history when many stories are being cut down to short social media posts, where communication has been reduced to emojis, and where the deep stories of our world, which can only be told by seasoned journalists, are disappearing, maybe it is time to sit down and share my own story of struggle and hope, suffering and laughter, anxiety and peace, and death and life. Maybe there is something in here that someone may find some strength in, something that someone can relate to. Maybe there is something in here that I can learn or have pointed out to me by someone else. Or maybe there is just something funny in here that can brighten your day and make you laugh. For as my wife, Kim, likes to joke, and as you will soon find out, I was not the brightest of kids!

Ultimately, I am hoping there is something here that can bind us together as human beings. There is something in the struggle for life that unites and inspires us, and maybe there is something in my story that can communicate that despite your own burdens, you are not alone. Most likely, life is not turning out the way you had planned. However, there is a new normal waiting just around the corner for you to step in to, and if something in my story can help you take that step, help you learn something that I missed in my own journey, or give you the courage to embrace what is next, then maybe this process of writing will be worth it in the end.

One final note. The story of my journey with cystic fibrosis and organ transplant is not meant to be prescriptive of other people's experience or current medical practices. In the eleven years since

Preface

I have received my transplant, things have changed considerably. This book is merely meant as a story of my own journey with CF and receiving a double-lung transplant. Every person who has CF, or who has undergone a lung-transplant, has their own unique experiences, and I presume to speak for no one else's experience but my own. This book is simply meant as an insight into my own journey with CF and transplantation and, hopefully, a narrative-companion for you in your own life-challenges.

Cheers.

INTRODUCTION

> "All we need to do is stop pounding
> on the door that just closed,
> turn around ... and welcome the
> largeness of life that now lies open."
>
> (*Let Your Life Speak*, Parker Palmer)

THE HEAVY AUTOMATIC doors swung open, and the two porters steered my stretcher through them. As we rounded the corner, I heard the doors bang closed behind us, separating me from my wife and parents.

A long, dim hallway stretched out before me. We had been waiting so long for this moment—days, weeks, months, years—but now that it was here and the clock was actually ticking, we didn't seem to have enough time. The porters picked up their pace from a brisk walk to a jog. We slid past state-of-the-art operating rooms, empty and silent at the late hour. Up ahead, I could see a set of open doors. Light spilled out of them into the cool, darkened hallway. *That must be it,* I thought.

As we approached the open doors, the porters slowed to a walk, and I got my first look at the shimmering, sanitized room in which the most pivotal moment of my life would take place. For some reason, in all my daydreams of what this day might look like, I'd

Big Breath In

never pictured the operating room. I'd thought endlessly about getting a double-lung transplant. For the last year and a half, the sole focus of my life had been my failing lungs. Lungs that, due to the fatal effects of cystic fibrosis (CF), were subject to raging, antibiotic-resistant bacterial infections. Lungs that were drowning in their own mucus. Lungs whose delicate airways were being sealed off by mounting scar tissue. My lungs now resembled two gray stones rather than pink elastic orbs. The effects of CF had suffocated them beyond resuscitation.

Over the previous eighteen months, I had replayed over and over again in my mind what this transplant day would look like. What I would say to my parents when the call came to tell me a set of lungs had become available. I pictured the ride to the hospital with my wife, Kim. The anticipation of waiting to be brought down from the ward, saying my goodbyes (you know, just in case), and giving Kim a last kiss. I had anticipated the bittersweetness of the day, feeling the excitement of what it could potentially mean for me—a new life—but also knowing the only reason I was getting a second chance at life was because a family somewhere else, probably not more than a half-day drive away, was saying their final goodbyes to their loved one. Their tragedy would lead to a miracle for me. But in all the mental preparation and dreaming of this day, I had never pictured this place: the operating room, ground zero of everything I had been waiting for!

What met my eyes as we left the dark hallway for the bright operating room was like something out of a movie set. The room would have been spacious if not for the multitude of machines, trays, tubes, and people who would keep me alive for the next eight hours or more. The smell of antibacterial clearing solutions filled my nostrils as a small army of nurses, technicians, and specialists bustled about preparing to do their job—to keep me alive as my naturally born lungs were removed from my body and replaced

Introduction

with lungs that only hours earlier were inflating and deflating inside the body of another person.

My bed came to a stop beside what looked like an overly large metal tray. The fact that it was in the center of the room with a very bright light hanging over it brought me to the conclusion that this would be my bed, the grand dissection tray for the medical professionals who would surround me tonight. I was helped onto the surgical table and lay down on my back. My oxygen tubing was transferred from the oxygen tank on the stretcher to the room's system. New intravenous bags were hung and hooked into the PICC line in my upper right arm. The stretcher I was brought in on was wheeled away, and the double doors through which I had arrived closed like a vault. I couldn't help but wonder if the closing of these doors had any greater significance. But there was no time for dark imagery now. This was it. It was now or never. Whatever the next hours would bring, I was at peace.

1.
CHILDHOOD

"It is by its content rather than
its duration that a child knows time,
by its quality rather than its quantity . . .
the place where I started out was Eden, of course.
One way or another it is where all of us start out,
if we have any luck at all."

(*The Sacred Journey,* Frederick Buechner)

I WAS BORN in 1982, the youngest of three children, to Art and Wilma Keulen. Both born in the mid-1950s, my parents are hardworking, salt-of-the-earth people, both the children of Dutch immigrants to the Fraser River Delta in the lowermost left-hand corner of Canada. Like all their parents before them, my parents are dairy farmers, and they took over the family farm that my grandpa (my dad's dad) started in the mid-1960s. My dad stands about six feet tall but is a little hunched from a lifetime of working with animals much larger than him that care little about the human body's fragilities. My mom stands at my shoulder height, and I am often told she looks incredibly young and fit for her age.

Along with my brother, Warren, and sister, Lynette, I spent my early days running and biking around our family farm, exploring the paths and laneways to our barns and fields. In the spring and summer, the three of us would take daily trips down the laneway behind the barns, over an abandoned railway track, and into a fallow field where grass grew taller than any child and trees grew in such a way that they looked like they could come alive at any moment (think *The Lord of the Rings*).

Each summer, my cousin Ken, who is a year older than me, would spend a week with me on the farm. We spent our days playing hockey, riding bikes, playing with our farm toys, and for some reason listening to Roxette's "Joyride" over and over again. (Damn, I miss the early '90s!) When not listening to Roxette on my sister's cassette player (yeah, that's right, I said "cassette player"), we would be outside, climbing trees, and letting our imaginations run wild. Trees normal to the adult eye would take the form of a large military bomber, naval destroyer, or anything with enough firepower to eliminate the imaginary enemy that dared cross the expanse of our childhood imaginations.

Warren

Though I was raised in a loving and joy-filled home, child-rearing came with a great deal of pain and heartbreak for my parents. Back in the 1970s, in their mid-twenties and with dreams of having a large family, my parents were unaware that the hereditary lineage each inherited from their respective family lines had some deadly anomalies in it. On their own, the recessive genes and anomalies they each carried were not a big deal, and they passed unnoticed down the family tree. However, when mixed with those of another person with the same recessive genetic mutations, this

Childhood

combination could create a genetic cocktail that no parent would ever dream of.

On March 19, 1977, my parents were overjoyed to welcome their first child, my older brother, Warren, into the world. Back then (and maybe still today), every farmer dreamed of having a child who might one day grow up and take over the family business.

A healthy, happy baby, Warren cooed and gurgled, cried and laughed like any other infant. But when he was about eight months of age, my parents noticed that something was not quite right in Warren's physical development. When most babies are starting to pull their chubby little legs underneath them and begin crawling, Warren would just kind of pull himself around with his arms, army crawling around the living room floor with his legs twitching behind him. When the time came for Warren to try walking, they could see that this weakness in his legs persisted. He seemed unable to pull his legs up under himself to support his own weight. After some doctors' appointments, waiting, testing, and then waiting some more, the diagnosis came back that Warren had spinal muscular atrophy.

Spinal muscular atrophy (SMA) is a genetic disorder that affects the voluntary muscles that are used for crawling, walking, head and neck control, and swallowing. People with SMA are often born with weak muscles, and those muscles continue to weaken and atrophy over time. Leg weakness is often more prominent than arm and hand weakness. The intellect of someone with SMA is, however, left unaffected. Oftentimes persons with SMA are exceptionally bright and thoughtful.

Over time, SMA can affect the respiratory muscles as well, thus leading to pneumonia and other severe chest infections with fatal consequences. In short, SMA is a fatal disease that eventually kills all children born with it, usually before they reach their mid-teens, and often in infancy.

What hopes and dreams my parents had of one day farming with their eldest son were shattered. Warren was sentenced to a life of body braces and living in a wheelchair with motor function only in his upper body. When it came down to it, my parents couldn't have cared less if Warren would ever be a farmer or not; all they wanted was that he be given as long a life as possible with as little suffering possible.

By the time of Warren's diagnosis, my mom was already pregnant with my older sister, Lynette. They were relieved to find that she was healthy and would not suffer the same life struggles as her older brother.

Lynette, even as a child, was a protector. Whenever Warren drove his wheelchair too close to a ditch or cow, Lynette would begin calling him back, urging him to be more careful. Later, when I came along, Lynette became like a supervisor for me, not allowing me out of her sight when we were outside. She could always be found with one hand on the back of Warren's wheelchair and the other hand holding my own, acting as conscience for any adventure we boys devised. This attitude of caregiver and protector has led Lynette into a career in critical care nursing (more on this later).

Four years after Lynette was born, I came sliding into the world. However, those four years of hope for another healthy child were dashed within days, as like my older brother, it was soon found that my genetic code also contained some fatal abnormalities, abnormalities known as cystic fibrosis. The writing was now on the wall that the inherited genetic makeup of our family was a game of Russian roulette. Like spinal muscular atrophy, cystic fibrosis profoundly changed the course of our family life.

Despite these early broken hearts, my parents were resilient in making our home a happy and as-normal-as-possible place to be. Looking back, I can see now that there was not a lot about our

Childhood

home life that most people would consider "normal." But it was the only life we knew, and we definitely made the most of it.

Because Warren used a wheelchair to get around, our house needed to be modified over time. Soon after Warren was old enough to drive his own electric wheelchair, a ramp needed to be installed to the back door of our house, and so my dad and grandpa got busy building and pouring a permanent concrete ramp onto the back of the house. The ramp had a 90-degree bend in it, extending from the back door and then turning outwards to the backyard, which of course made it awesome for riding my bike down.

Because of Warren's chair, we always owned vans. Whenever a new van was purchased (which rarely ever happened because, don't forget, we are a Dutch family), Dad and Grandpa would go to work ripping out the rear bench seat and installing hooks to anchor Warren's wheelchair while we drove.

Warren was fearless. The van we owned during my childhood was a 1983 Dodge Ram. This was no minivan that was low to the ground with an automatic lift in it; this was a campervan that my dad modified himself.

Whenever we would go somewhere, my parents, sister, or I (when I was old enough) would open the back barn-doors of the van and pull out the two skinny metal ramps that a local agricultural-equipment fabricator made for us. Sometimes, before the ramps were even hooked securely in place, Warren would go flying up them into the back of the van. Then, to get out, he would whip his wheelchair around in the van, and whether the ramps were hooked in or just sitting on the bumper, he would come flying down those skinny strips of metal and be off to wherever he needed to be.

My dad would also install seat belts on the rear wheel-wells, and this is where I would often sit, right beside my big brother, my knees knocking into the side of his chair whenever we turned a corner. Because it was just the metal of the wheel-well that I was sitting on with no seat cushion or anything, it tended to get a bit cold in the rainy winter, but it was a fun place to sit. I should say, this wasn't child abuse or anything; there was still a nice comfortable bench seat in front of where my brother was anchored and where my parents always told me to sit. But as a kid who looked up to and admired his older brother, it was just much more fun to sit with him in the back of the van, even if it meant feeling the ping of every rock that the wheel picked up on the road. Lynette, being older and the family protector, usually sat on the factory-installed comfortable bench seat.

When it came time for family vacations, we didn't miss a beat. When Warren's wheelchair became too big to fit into the side door of our family motorhome, my dad took the motorhome to a mechanic, who cut a larger door in the side so Warren could once again drive right on up into it. He would again be anchored to hooks my dad installed and would sit between the driver and passenger, following along on the map and taking in all the miles we put on.

Many other places that Warren frequented needed to be equipped with ramps as well. It is commonplace today to see ramps in most public buildings, but back in the late '70s and early '80s, there was not a lot of disability awareness, especially spinal disabilities and injuries, so it was very difficult for people in wheelchairs to get around.

Locally, in Vancouver, Rick Hansen has become the face and muscle behind physical disability awareness and advocacy. Back in 1973, when Rick was fifteen years old, he was involved in a car accident on a rural road on the way back from a fishing trip. He was thrown from the back of the pickup truck he was riding in, suffering a spinal cord injury that paralyzed him from the waist down. Soon after the injury, Rick began playing wheelchair sports and participating in wheelchair marathon races. In 1985, he began his *Man in Motion World Tour*, in which he wheeled his chair around the world, raising awareness for disabilities and accessibility. He completed his world tour in just over two years, raising over $26 million for spinal cord injury research and rehabilitation. This, however, was still years away from where Warren and my parents found themselves. Therefore, ramps had to be installed at our elementary school and church, and both sets of grandparents also installed permanent concrete ramps outside their homes.

This was no doubt a painful process for my parents, with each ramp a reminder of how different Warren was and the unique challenges he had to face in his young life. As I reflect now, and I think of all those ramps our family installed in homes, our school, and our church, they were all permanent fixtures to these buildings. Even though the adults knew the mortal challenge facing Warren, these ramps were never installed with the thought that they would one day be taken down when Warren passed—they would be there forever with the expectation and hope that Warren would be as well. Built strong and permanent, they stood as a testament to the love and respect shown to Warren, even if it was our family who had to advocate to get these done. Warren was loved by many in our larger community, and many hands pitched in to help with these projects, but it took Warren and his chair to show how far we as a community, and society as a whole, were from being inclusive of people who were differently abled. I see now how Warren, my parents, and my grandparents really were trailblazers of inclusivity in our community.

The most unique modification to our house was an elevator we had installed in 1987. Again, it was mainly my dad, grandpa, and employees on our farm who did most of the work for this. The elevator was not installed because of the size of our house—we lived in a modest two-story farmhouse—but once Warren reached the age of nine, it was getting more difficult for my parents to carry him up and down the steep staircase to his bedroom, along with this heavier chair. It was essential to my parents that Warren be able to go everywhere in the house that anyone else could go, so the idea of him not being able to go upstairs and have a bedroom where all of our bedrooms were was out of the question. And so, after Expo 86 in Vancouver, my parents bought an industrial freight elevator from the site and installed it in our house.

    Though Warren could never play conventional sports, he loved to watch them. Growing up, he learned everything he could about hockey and his favorite team, the Vancouver Canucks. Once I was old enough, he began imparting his knowledge to me, coaching me in the garage and on the driveway as I ran around his wheelchair with a hockey stick and ball. Often, Warren, Lynette, and I would go outside to play hockey in the yard. Lynette would give Warren his hockey stick, the upper part of which he would rest under his left armpit, running the shaft of the stick down between his legs and through the metal foot supports of his chair, and laying his left hand over the stick for stability. When the ball came toward Warren, he would line his chair up at a ninety-degree angle to the ball, square off to the goal, and at the last second, jerk the joystick of his chair, thus swinging it around so that the blade of the stick would contact the ball perfectly. He would actually get a pretty good shot off the majority of the time. Of course, he would also go and track down any stray ball his stupid younger brother would fire the wrong way, shooting it back to me, waiting docile near the net. Whenever Warren tired of playing, or when his electric wheelchair motor would heat up too much, or its battery would die down too far, he would park his chair on the side of the yard and coach Lynette and I while we slapped the ball around.

Warren also played wheelchair soccer. It is like regular soccer, except the ball is much larger, it is played in a gym, and each chair is outfitted with a bumper in order to "kick" the ball. It was very exciting to go to his games and see him complete, and also see the level of competition displayed at these tournaments. It was here that Warren was also able to connect with other people in wheelchairs, which was a very special thing. Warren, nor my parents, ever let his wheelchair slow him down. Yes, things looked different, but whether it was school, sports, or vacations, Warren knew what he wanted and always found a way to participate.

Growing up, Warren had a variety of wheelchairs. Just like kids wear out their running shoes, Warren would wear and grow out of his chairs. Because I was five years younger than him, I really only remember his last chair. It was a chrome-plated metal chair. It had four black tires all the same size. Its seat, arm, back, and headrest were all black, and at the end of the right armrest was a control console, with a joystick and a couple of other buttons that could control the lights and power on/off the TV. The battery and motor cover were white and sat underneath and behind his seat. The chair also had two handgrip bars sticking out from the backrest that one could use to push or pull the chair if the battery died, and from which Warren's backpack would usually hang. But the thing that I thought was coolest about the chair was that the seat could swivel around to the side. You could swing the seat 90 degrees from the front of the chair, so when the chair went forward, you could be sitting sideways. At the time, this concept of mechanics blew my little mind away!

After school, my mom would often lift Warren out of this chair, and he would rest on the couch and watch TV. This is when I would seize my opportunity. Ever since I can remember, I have always loved driving, and Warren's chair was the first taste I got of it. As soon as Warren was taken out of his chair and my mom went to the other room, I was all over it!

If you were to have walked through our house during our childhood years, you would have seen many banged-up doorframes, missing paint chips from the walls and doors about a foot from the floor, and many scrapes on the kitchen cabinets. These were not caused by Warren—well, maybe some of them were—but the majority were caused by me. Warren was an excellent driver. Patient, careful, and obviously experienced, rarely did he run into a wall, scrape a doorframe, or drive over any toes. I, on the other hand, didn't really care.

Because I was not allowed to take the chair outside or use the elevator to take the chair upstairs, I did most of my damage downstairs. Often, my little joy rides would end with my being scolded by my mom, Warren, or Lynette. (Come on, Lynette!) Or, on a couple of occasions, they ended with me draining the battery, leaving Warren on the couch for most of the evening and me cowering in my room, waiting for the reprimand I knew was coming once one of my parents found the incapacitated chair somewhere it wasn't supposed to be. (Yes, I was an inconsiderate little shit.)

The End of Eden

Like most people, I remember a lot of firsts in my life. The first time I learned to tie my shoes, the first time I took the bus home from school, my first day of high school, the first day I got my license, my first kiss (and I mean real kiss, not the silly elementary schoolyard pecks), and the first time I wanted my good-friend-Kim to be *more* than just my good-friend-Kim. However, the greatest impact any "first" has had on me was the first time I experienced the death of a person I loved.

Childhood

In the spring of 1991, much of the early childhood fun and happiness drained from our home. Summer 1990, following surgery to put a metal rod in Warren's back to help him sit up straighter in his chair, doctors discovered his lung function and respiratory muscles had atrophied, quite unnoticed, to a critical level. My parents were told that any kind of cold or flu could quickly turn into pneumonia in Warren's weakened lungs and could prove fatal for him.

Over the fall, winter, and early spring of 1990 to 1991, my mom fought valiantly to protect Warren from the colds and flus that menacingly roamed our childhood environment, but in early April, the reality of Warren's genetic life sentence proved too much. Over two weeks during the end of March and early April, Warren caught a cold that developed into pneumonia. He was admitted to BC Children's Hospital and courageously fought for four long days. At 2:00 p.m. on April 10, 1991, Warren passed away.

Many of the details surrounding Warren's death are a blur to me, but there are some pockets of memory: getting into my grandparents' car after we were told to come to the hospital and the absolute silence of that hot, springtime ride. Walking from the elevator to Warren's hospital room in BC Children's Hospital. Running my right hand along the plastic railing on the wall. Turning the final corner around the nurse's station and seeing my uncle standing in the hallway outside Warren's room talking on the phone with tears in his eyes. Walking into Warren's room and seeing my silent parents looking longingly at their firstborn. Kissing Warren's cold forehead. Seeing his wheelchair in the corner of the room, empty.

I remember there were a lot of people at our house when we got home that afternoon, and that I hated the way I felt inside. Everyone seemed to bring food, most of which I found disgusting. One of our farm employees brought his son over to play with me and get me out of the house—I don't remember what we did, but I was thankful he was there.

Being in the house over the following days and weeks was difficult for everyone. Every once in a while, I caught my parents with tears in their eyes, whispering to each other, trying to hide the sorrow and tears from my sister and me. It was very quiet. The feeling that I felt as a nine-year-old was not so much one of sorrow—it would take years to fully understand the depth of loss and sorrow—but rather of discomfort. I didn't like seeing everyone crying; I didn't like how I felt; I didn't like it when people were sad.

There is not a lot I remember of the funeral. Most of the things I remember were things that simply affected me. I remember being excited to ride in a limo, but then being disappointed when I was told I had to ride up front with the driver because there was not enough room in the back. In retrospect, it was probably for the best, as the driver was a very friendly woman who tried to keep my mind occupied with other things. Looking back, I can't imagine the weight of sorrow that must have filled the back of that limo, with my parents, sister, and grandparents back there, all knowing they were being driven to say their final goodbye to their brother, son, grandchild.

To this day, I still shudder when I think of the further grief I may have caused my parents due to insensitive comments, trying to live like nothing had happened, trying to cheer my parents up, and not fully grasping the weight of sorrow and loss my parents were experiencing.

My parents went to great lengths to put on a brave face and hide their grief from me over the following weeks, months, and even years. In my later teens, my sister shared the true extent of what they went through. I can only stand in awe at the depth of strength and character my parents have, shielding me as best they could from the darkness and trauma they were living.

Over time, our home returned to the warm and happy place it had been, but there was always something different. A large piece of our family was torn away from us, and a wound as deep as that never fully heals. A scar formed over the grief, but it was one that could be ripped open without a moment's notice. Our grief was not always obvious to the naked eye, but it hid in the corners of our life together, and still does, manifesting itself in unpredictable ways, or when an insensitive comment is made by a well-meaning but oblivious person, and of course during significant times of the year.

I include Warren's story here not just because it is a part of my life, but because Warren's life and death have emotional reverberations on the way we as a family faced my genetic challenges and mortality many years later.

Warren passed away decades ago, but his fourteen years of life, and his death, are still etched deep into my parents, sister, and me. It has shaped us into the people we are today. It has created a strength and understanding that we share, but it has also created a brokenness. It has created incredible resiliency in each of us, but it has also set strict emotional boundaries.

Warren's life and death cemented a stability, empathy, and wisdom in my parents I have yet to experience in anyone else in my life.

For my sister, it created a single-minded drive to care for the sick, to be with and care for those in mortal crisis; to want to be with the sickest of the sick and nurse back to health those on the brink of death—and to be incredibly calm and caring while doing so.

And for me, Warren's life and death has impacted me more than I am probably even aware of, but most important for this story, it created a self-imposed mantle that I would not become the second child that my parents would bury due to a fatal genetic illness. When the time came for me to fight for my own life, it was not so much for myself that I fought, or even for my wife, but it was for my parents—flawed genetics were not going to win this time.

It was Warren, in his life and death, who gave me the strength and determination to fight the long fight when I needed to. It was his life, taken too soon, that gave me the determination to fight for a second chance at mine.

2.
EARLY LIFE WITH CYSTIC FIBROSIS

"Even when a cure is impossible,
healing is not necessarily impossible.
While medical science has limits, hope does not."
(*The Lost Art of Healing,* Bernard Lown, MD)

I WAS BORN in uneventful fashion on February 26, 1982. Though my parents named my brother after my grandpa, and my sister after my *oma* (my mom's mom), I was given the name George—my dad just always wanted a "George."

Though my birth was routine, what followed in the coming days was anything but. Three days after I was born, it was discovered that I had a meconium ileus. Basically put, a meconium ileus is a blockage of the bowel. No big deal, right? Well, in terms of surgery and procedure, yes, no big deal. However, a meconium ileus is often the first symptom of something much more menacing. A bright and quick-thinking nurse was the first to make the connection between my bowel blockage and the fact this could be a sign of something far more serious. At three days old, I underwent surgery, leaving me with a large, grotesque scar across my belly. To confirm if the blockage was a sign of something more sinister, as the nurse suspected, I was also administered a sweat test, the standard diagnostic tool for cystic fibrosis. This test is exactly what it sounds like: a test to measure the amount of sodium and chloride in my sweat. Elevated levels of these elements in the sweat signal something deadly. My test results came back positive—enter our family's second chronic fatal illness: cystic fibrosis. Once again, my parents' dreams of having a healthy baby boy were dashed on the hospital room floor, and they were again left wondering what kind of quality and quantity of life their son would have.

Cystic fibrosis (CF) is a genetic illness affecting the lungs, liver, pancreas, intestines, bowel, sinuses, and reproductive system—it has ramifications for almost every part of the body. But, in most cases, the most damaging effects are on the lungs. A recessive gene causes CF; thus, both parents need to be carrying the gene. When this is the case, a child has a 25% chance of having full-blown CF. Many people, especially of Western European descent, are unknowingly carriers of the CF gene.

Everyone has a thin layer of water and mucus in their lungs to help filter out particles in the air we breathe. However, for people with CF, the mucus that is supposed to protect our airways is thicker and stickier, with much more of it than there should be. Thus, over time, the mucus plugs the airways in the lungs and provides a perfect environment for bacteria to get caught and begin reproducing, which causes severe respiratory infections. Each infection causes scarring to the lung tissue, thus hardening and killing it, reducing lung capacity and airflow. Over time, and with enough infections and airway scarring, there is essentially not enough good lung tissue left to survive. The life of the person with CF is choked out of them. Incredible research into gene mapping, genetic mutations, and treatment for CF has taken place over the past three decades, but still, over half the people who die from CF in Canada every year die before they reach the age of thirty.

With my birth and diagnosis, my parents were once again thrown into the role of parents and caregivers. As my dad was a self-employed dairy farmer, and as farming is a 24/7 kind of vocation, my mom took charge of my health by making sure she knew all she could about CF and how to care for a child with it.

It was paramount to my parents that I remain as healthy as possible, but along with that was their desire that I not be seen as *different*. Warren had lived with a disability that was very public. He had no choice—a child couldn't stick out more than Warren did. Whether we were at school, the mall, or on vacation, kids would simply stop and stare at Warren, and though adults would try to be more discrete and sensitive, they would often stare just as hard as their kids. This experience was not something my parents wanted me to have to go through as well.

Because I was healthy throughout my childhood, we were able to keep my CF diagnosis under wraps. My parents did not go to great lengths to do this, but because I was healthy and could often excel at many sports and activities, it was easy to keep a lid on the fact that, like my brother, I also suffered from a fatal genetic illness. No parent wants to see their child singled out as different, and because my CF was uncharacteristically mild as a child, I was lucky not to be, at least not outside my own terms.

This meant that when I was outside the house—at school, with friends, or playing ice hockey—I had the same opportunities as other kids. My parents always knew what I was up to, and if it didn't present a great risk to my health, then any activity was fair game. But when we got home, it was treatment time!

Regular treatment for my CF involved respiratory physiotherapy that took place twice a day, pills that had to be taken with every meal, and a vigilant watch for any respiratory infection that might be brewing in my lungs. However, having this be part of my daily life since before I can remember, I didn't give the inconvenience and "different-ness" of it too much thought at this point. All these medical things were just part of my regular day-to-day routine.

My mom, who trained and worked as a registered nurse before having kids, and who had already spent countless hours in clinics and doctors' offices with Warren, was a veteran when it came to dealing with my doctors and clinic visits. I would often sit passively as my mom pushed doctors for more treatment and clearer explanations of what was happening with my lungs, demanding that even though I was healthier than many children with CF, our concerns still be taken seriously.

CF Clinic and Physiotherapy

Every three months, I had an appointment at the CF clinic at BC Children's Hospital. As a child, I never minded going there. The only problem was the waiting. For me, going to the clinic meant a half-day off from school, and sometimes, if my mom got frustrated and we had to wait an extra-long time for a test or to see the doctor, that half-day became a whole day off.

The CF clinic was on the ground floor of the Hospital. When I attended clinic, before the days of strict infection control, us CF kids and our parents all sat together in a large waiting room. (It is widely known today that due to transmission of respiratory infections, people with CF should not be in close quarters with each other.) On the other side of the administration desk was another large room with four cubicles in it, and with doctors' offices and exam rooms exiting off on three sides. Through the large room and farther down a long hallway was the pulmonary function lab, and one floor up was the blood lab and X-ray area.

Early Life with Cystic Fibrosis

During those half-day clinic visits, which happened every three months, it never occurred to me how hard it must have been for my mom to keep going back to that hospital, as it was the exact place where Warren had died, just three floors up from where my clinic was. I can't imagine the strength of character and brave face she must have had to put on each time we parked in the same parking lot and walked through those sliding glass doors where she had also brought my brother so many times before.

My clinic visits always included a pulmonary function test (PFT). The PFT involves breathing into a machine three times, then taking a *BIG BREATH IN*, and then blowing out all the air in your lungs until there is nothing left. The test measures lung capacity and functionality of the airways. It is a hellish test to continually do. At clinic, I would get an X-ray done once a year. Twice a year, I would cry or at least sniffle my way through bloodwork (and one time I vomited). Each visit would include meeting with the CF-specialized nurse, a dietician, a social worker, and a physiotherapist. I would need my throat swabbed each visit, almost bringing me to the point of vomiting (again) to see which bacteria I was growing in my airways. Each visit ended by meeting with the doctor. My mom shared with me that when I was a small child, each clinic visited also included a major meltdown and inconsolable temper tantrum. All of this usually took about three hours (the clinic, not the tantrum).

The best part of the clinic visits was after we were done, my mom and I would stop at the hospital cafeteria, and I could get a large raisin-bran muffin and either chocolate-milk or pop. These were always a treat for me. If the visit had gone well and things with my health were looking up, or if my mom had been able to distract herself from the reality of what this hospital represented to her, she was good company and we would talk about things we saw or maybe about certain hockey games I had coming up.

But if things had not gone well with the doctors or the memory of Warren haunted her more than other times, we would sit in silence in the cafeteria, me munching obliviously on my raisin-bran muffin with my chocolate milk or pop.

Other than taking a handful of pills every time I would eat, the most intrusive part of CF was the twice a day physiotherapy treatments. Until the mid-1990s, the most effective physiotherapy treatment for CF patients was percussion physio. This involves the patient, me, laying stomach-down on my mom's lap and having her literally beat the mucus out of my lungs. Of course, it was not as bad as it sounds. It was a simple, rhythmic drumming on my back, then on my sides, and then on my chest itself. The primary purpose of percussion physio is to get the clogged mucus to move up the airways where it can be coughed out of the lungs. After doing percussions in each position for about five minutes, I would sit up and do some huffing. (Huffing is like it sounds, just put a lot of energy and emphasis on the "h" sound.) I would then try to cough up any mucus the beating and huffing had loosened!

It is a time-consuming treatment and would usually last about twenty to thirty minutes each morning and evening. For me, it was not a big deal as I got to lay there and watch TV (*Power Rangers*, *Duck Tales*, and *Don Cherry's Rock'em Sock'em Hockey* were some of my favorites) and listen for my mom's instruction on when to sit up, huff, and cough.

As I mentioned earlier, my parents tried hard to make sure I had as normal a life as possible, and in public, this was so. The only time physio was a stark reminder for me of how different I was, and how much CF did actually interfere with life, was when we would go on road trips with my ice hockey team. Laying across my mom's lap, perched on the side of a hotel bed while I could hear my teammates running and yelling up and down the hallways without me was always difficult. At that time, that was the closest my private life of physiotherapy ever came to intersecting with my "normal" public childhood life.

There was, however, the taking of pancreatic enzymes. Most CF sufferers cannot digest their food properly because of damage done to their pancreas. Because of this, most CF patients need to take oral pancreatic enzymes whenever they want to eat something. When I went to school, my mom would roll a couple of enzyme pills in tin foil and pack them in my lunch. In this way, I learned responsibility at a very young age—I was an oblivious kid, but I was responsible. Whenever I didn't take my enzymes, I would be subject to nasty stomach cramps, and diarrhea would often be sure to follow the next day. Therefore, I learned in a hurry the importance of taking these gel capsule pills. The ridiculous thing is that even though I have taken oral enzymes every time I have eaten a meal in my whole life, there are still times today when I will leave the house, knowing I will be eating out, and forget my enzymes! When I was a child and teenager, my mom would always carry extra pills for me in her purse, and truth be told, embarrassing as it is, my wife does this now too.

There would often be other pills added to my daily regimen of enzymes. A couple of times a year, my mom would tell me it was time to take antibiotics because I was showing signs of a chest infection, but I never paid much attention to these things. If my mom told me to take this or that white or pink pill, it was okay with me; she knew what she was talking about.

Antibiotics are a life-saving and regular part of life for people with CF. I was very lucky not to need intravenous antibiotics like so many other kids with CF, as this would have landed me in the hospital often. My chest infections could always be kept under control with a regimen of oral antibiotics, usually lasting for two weeks at a time.

Big Breath In

Being active is another important health factor for people with CF. Any medium to vigorous activity helps strengthen the lung muscles, but it also helps move the suffocating mucus higher into the airways where it can be coughed out easier. Luckily for me, I was always a very active child and teenager. Growing up on a farm, one tends to grow up running and biking all over the place. Whenever a friend came over, it was imperative that they brought their bike with them. Much of my after-school time and weekends was spent riding around and around our farm or over to a friend's house, who lived on a neighboring farm.

When I was seven years old, my parents enrolled me in ice hockey. Now, everything I knew about ice hockey I had learned from my brother, Warren, but being in a wheelchair, the one thing he could not do was teach me was how to skate, and I was brutal at it!

I remember the first time I got on the ice and had my first session of power skating. It was an hour of skating with other kids my age to help make you into a better skater. For me, it was not so much about being a better skater as it was about learning how to skate altogether. I was late for my very first session. My mom tied my skates, put my helmet on my head, and did up the chin strap. She then opened the door to the ice surface and sent me out. I spent my very first five minutes on the ice crying in front of the door that was now closed behind me as I wanted to get off the ice so badly. My mom—knowing that there were going to be many times in life when, for the sake of my health, and survival, I would need to face my fears and push through them—stood on the other side of the glass with my sister and refused to open the door. She just pointed to the open ice behind me.

Though I hated those first couple sessions of skating, as an adult looking back, I am so thankful that my mom never opened the gate to let me off the ice. She knew the courage and independence

I was going to need to develop in order make it in this life with CF. There have been many times in my health struggles where I have wanted to hide, wanted to quit, wanted to turn back time and return to what was safe and familiar, but of course, I couldn't. Learning to face my fears at a young age, learning to turn around from the familiar and build up the courage to face the unknown, even with tears in my eyes, was the most important thing that would get me through some of the challenges I would later face.

After getting through those first sessions of power skating, it was time for team tryouts. Now when I say tryouts, it is not the kind of thing that pops into most people's heads. At this young age, tryouts are just practice drills that all the kids go through so the coaches can watch and then together split everyone into teams, with each team having an equal share of the talent pool (me treading in the shallow end of that pool).

These tryouts involved pucks, which was a new thing for me. I remember getting on the ice early, finding a puck, and shooting it down the ice. I would then skate as fast as I could, loose ankles splayed out 45-degrees to the ice, chasing the puck down. After reaching the puck, I would turn around, shoot it to the other end of the rink, and once again go chasing after it. After watching me do this a couple of times, one coach skated over and told me to keep the puck on my stick as I skated instead of always shooting it ahead of me.

I loved playing hockey, but I was not a natural skater or scorer. There was, however, one position that came naturally to me, and that was goalie. People always say you need to be a bit crazy to be a goalie, and I guess that glove fit me! The thing that first drew me to goaltending was the equipment. I've always been a gearhead; the big pads, the big glove, and the blocker—that was the stuff! It was also the idea that the goalie was one-of-a-kind, a lone wolf on the ice, though I do enjoy working in groups. (Okay, I actually don't enjoy working in groups; I don't know why I wrote that. I have never enjoyed working in groups, but I always feel bad when I say this, like I'm antisocial or something . . . okay, maybe I *am* a bit antisocial). I have always preferred to work alone. I also enjoy working under pressure. All these factors made the idea of being a goalie irresistible to me, much to my mom's chagrin. My parents put me in ice hockey in order to be active and to get some good winter exercise; standing in one spot for half the game was not their idea of activity. But after much persistence, and seeing and hearing that I actually had a bit of a natural talent for it, she relented and I became a goalie.

Over the next couple years, I improved my skill and began playing in the top level for my age group. While playing on more competitive teams, this also meant more ice time and a lot more travel. By the time I was twelve and thirteen years old, we were on the ice six times a week and usually traveling somewhere in the province once a month. This began to take a toll at home and on the farm. My parents and I decided that when I started high school, I would stop playing for the city and instead join a recreational church league that many of my friends were already playing in. Hockey was no longer fun, and it was time I started directing my life toward other things. I also decided I no longer wanted to play goalie. I wanted to actually be more social, and I was beginning to see that being an active player was good for me.

Joining the rec league did not mean that my competitive hockey days were over. In fact, if you know anything about church leagues, they can be some of the most competitive, not skilled, but competitively violent leagues around! I don't know what it was—if it was because we were all made to sit in church every Sunday morning or told to always be "good little boys"—but when we stepped on the ice, something happened, and all the pent-up teenage energy and "evilness" seemed to rise to the surface and come striding out!

Adolescent Years

It was around this time, aged thirteen or so, that I became more aware that I differed from those around me. CF was becoming more of a reality in my life. Now, this did not have so much to do with worsening symptoms or anything, although I was noticing myself coughing more; it had more to do with entering the age of growing self-awareness.

During my childhood, it was always my brother, Warren, who was the sick one. Most of our family's health attention focused his way. Sure, I took pills every time I ate and my mom did percussion chest physio on me every day, but I was still healthy and could do everything any other boy my age could do, and when it came to sports, I could often excel. But now, as I reached high-school age, I was seeing that I also had some differences.

In the years since Warren had passed away, life had developed a new normal around our house and farm. I was taking on new levels of independence, and with that independence came new levels of responsibility. It was no longer my mom who was solely responsible for my care and well-being, but I was now expected to step up to the plate. I was the one who needed to remember to take my pancreatic enzymes before meals. If my mom noticed that I'd forgotten, she would remind me at the last second, but I was now taking more responsibility for my own body and illness.

The ways of doing physiotherapy also changed around this time. The early and mid-1990s had seen some big jumps in CF research, and one of these jumps had to do with the way youth and adults could undertake more independent forms of physiotherapy.

Chest percussions were being replaced by new inhaled nebulized medications and other breathing mask apparatuses. My mom, knowing that chest percussions were a tried and trusted way of airway clearance, was a little hesitant on trying these new techniques. After all, why change something that isn't broken? But as I ventured into my adolescent years, trying to create a sense of independence, I was getting a little self-conscious and sheepish about having to every day, sometimes twice a day, lay down on my mom's lap or sit on the floor in front of her and have her try to beat the mucus out of my lungs. Therefore, I welcomed these new physiotherapy innovations.

The first new technique we tried was called the PEP mask. PEP stands for positive expiratory pressure. The mask that I used was a three-piece device. The first part was the face mask, which was cone-shaped and made of hard, clear plastic. On the large open end of the mask there was a fitted rubber edge that fit around my nose and mouth so that all my breathing would be done through the mask. It is like a mask a pilot would wear when flying a jet, just a lot smaller. On the outward-facing end of the mask was a hole that would attach to a three-inch-long hollow T-shaped piece of hard plastic. On the other end of the T was a one-way value. This valve would allow air into the mask when you took a breath in but would not allow air out. On the bottom of the T-shape, an air restrictor was attached. Depending on the age and air capacity of the patient, the restrictor would be different sizes, usually measured in millimeters.

The concept of the mask was that the patient breathed in through the one-way valve, which then closed, thus forcing the person to exhale all the air out of their lungs through the small restrictor hole. This technique helped create strong respiratory muscles, but the real effect was that it created positive pressure within the lungs, thus forcing oxygen deep down into the smaller airways that were often partially blocked with mucus buildup or scar tissue. The therapy would get oxygen in behind the scar tissue and mucus and thus begin moving that mucus up and into the larger airways where it could then be huffed and coughed out.

This mask represented not just a new way of doing respiratory physio, but it also gave CF patients a new sense of freedom and independence. As I was an adolescent when I began using this new devise, it symbolized a further step in taking responsibility and ownership of my health. No longer was I the passive patient sitting idle while my mom tried to beat the CF out of me. I now had to do some real work and had to develop some new disciplines. My mom would still keep a close supervising eye on what I was doing, reminding me to pay attention to my form and the effort I was putting in. I had to remain focused on my technique and count my breaths so I knew when to stop breathing through the PEP mask and try huffing and coughing, but overall, this new form of physio seemed to work out well.

Every morning, I would get up at 7:00 a.m. and head downstairs. The first part of my morning physiotherapy was my PEP mask. I would take two hits of Ventolin from my puffer and grab my mask, which was usually in a Tupperware container in the kitchen. Using the PEP mask was not just a matter of sitting there and breathing in and out, although I admit this is what it often turned into for me and my distracted mind. Proper technique involved taking fifteen breaths in and out, then taking the mask off and doing a series of huffs and coughs to try to bring up any mucus that the positive pressure may have brought higher in the airways. Of course, I would often lose focus and forget how many breaths I had taken. I would then repeat this six times.

Every couple of years, as researchers kept improving the PEP mask, I ended up adding more attachment to it. Instead of taking Ventolin through the traditional puffer, I attached a nebulizer cup to it. This cup attached to the end of the PEP mask, and I attached the bottom of the cup to plastic tubing attached to a small air compressor. The machine pumped air into this small cup containing liquid Ventolin, turning the liquid into a vapor to be breathed in for the duration of the physiotherapy exercise.

After doing PEP for about 20 minutes, which is roughly the time it took to use up all the Ventolin, I put the mask (and now the nebulizer cup too) back on the counter for my mom to clean (yes, I was that kind of teenager) and I would prepare my next drug. If I had an active chest infection, I would often then be put on an inhaled antibiotic. This was also a nebulized drug that came in a large bottle, and I would need to measure it out with a syringe. I would pull the proper amount of medication out of the bottle, squirt it into a new nebulizer cup, and attach that cup to a regular mask, which covered my nose and mouth. I would then sit on the couch again, breathing in this new vaporized medicine. Taking this sort of medication was easier than the PEP mask. I could just sit on the couch and not have to count my breaths. This was a drug I needed only once a day, and it usually took about ten minutes before all the liquid was vaporized. I would then put this mask with its empty nebulizer cup on the counter beside my PEP mask and go back to the fridge one more time for the third and final phase of my morning physio. This third phase of physio involved quite an expensive nebulized medication called Pulmozyme.

Pulmozyme is a very popular nebulized medication for people who have CF. I took it after all the other physio treatments because it is a longer-acting medication. Like the Ventolin and inhaled antibiotic, the liquid is vaporized in a nebulizer cup and breathed in. It acts in the lungs throughout the next number of hours, breaking up the mucus chunks in the airways. You want this medication to sit down in the lungs and work over whatever mucus is still down there that you weren't able to bring up during the use of the PEP mask or the other medications. To breathe in all the medication, which I found to have a distinct metallic taste, usually took around fifteen minutes. After finishing this last phase of my physiotherapy treatment, I would now be into my second half hour of morning TV shows.

From start to finish, my morning physio would usually take around 40 minutes. After this, my day looked like any other child or teenager's day, other than the five to eight pills I needed to take with each meal to help digest my food.

This was a routine that repeated itself every morning before school. Sometimes, when I was feeling great, I could skip my physio either on Saturday or Sunday morning. In the evenings, I would have to use my PEP mask again, but this time without the Ventolin.

Now maybe you're thinking, "How horrible, what a way to begin each day of your life!" And yes, you are right. Seven days a week, 365 days a year, this is the reality for most children, youth, and adults with CF, with some variations. However, for me at this age, it didn't seem like much of an inconvenience, as this was all I ever knew. I didn't know what it was like to sleep in, or to roll out of bed, grab a bowl of cereal and be off for the bus. Forty minutes of physiotherapy was all this kid knew about starting a day, so at the time it was not that big of a burden.

A funny story from a friend of mine who also has CF illustrates this point well. When he told my wife and me this story, my wife couldn't stop laughing because it reminded her so much of my lack of awareness as a child. Paul is a guy I met in 2012, after my transplant. He also has had a double-lung transplant. When Paul was about six years old, he had a next-door neighbor named Trevor. In the summer, Paul and Trevor played together every day, but being a kid with CF, Paul had to go through the whole physiotherapy routine with his mom every morning—30 minutes of percussion physio (this was still the days before PEP). Often, in the middle of Paul's physio treatment, his friend Trevor would come knocking on the door, poke his head inside, and ask when Paul could come out and play. Paul's mom always said, "In about 15 minutes, Trevor."

Finally, after a couple of weeks of this, Paul got frustrated that he was always stuck inside in the morning while Trevor was already outside playing. After one long session of physiotherapy and Trevor poking his head in the back door, Paul sat up from his mom's lap and protested, "Why does my physio always take so much longer than Trevor's?" Trevor, of course, didn't have CF. Physio had always been a regular part of Paul's life, like my own, that he couldn't imagine a morning routine that didn't involve laying down on your mom's lap and having her beat mucus out of your lungs. He just thought that all kids did physio and, for some aggravating reason, Trevor's physio was a lot shorter than his! When Paul told my wife and I this story, I couldn't help laughing, not laughing at him, but laughing at myself because of how much this story resonated with me.

Every morning, there are thousands of children, youth, and adults all across this country who get up and engage in a physio regimen such as my own before I had my transplant. Many kids and adults do much more than I did, and a few do less. But physio is a necessity of life for someone with CF. It is the first defense against the onslaught of mucus that is forever building up in the airways, waiting for some nasty bacteria to float into its grasp and to cause the next infection, leading to more lung tissue scaring. This is the vicious cycle of CF—mucus, bacteria, infection, scaring; mucus, bacteria, infection, scaring—over and over again, hardening the lungs and cutting off the airways.

This is why physiotherapy and airway clearance are so important. Patients need to keep the upper hand on the amount of mucus that sits in their lungs. Keeping it moving and getting it out are vital to the survival of a person with CF.

When an infection flares, physio time increases to at least three times a day. For children and youth who use PEP, a parent will also often begin chest percussions again to ensure the best results—anything to get the infected mucus up and out of the lungs. Physiotherapy is a matter of life and death. However, even with these defenses—physio, antibiotics, concerned loved ones and teams of health-care professionals coaching us on—the truth about CF is that no matter how many battles you fight against invading infections, each person with CF at some point comes to the awareness that CF is not so much a battle, but a war. A war of attrition that we are always losing.

3.
BECOMING AWARE

"He tends his flock like a shepherd:
He gathers the lambs in his arms"

(Isaiah 40:11 NIV)

LIVING WITH CF involves going to great lengths to protect and monitor your physical health. Exercise, physio, antibiotics, vitamins, and a whole array of other treatments and pills become part of life, and they are always changing. One's treatment of one's CF is a continual learning curve. However, this learning curve is not restricted to one's physical health. The mental and emotional learning curve, and the ever-constant evolution of one's self-awareness, is also a long journey that one needs to navigate if one wants to be as healthy as possible. And it is often, once the child has taken more responsibility for their physical health, that they then also begin to traverse the land of learning what some of these physical barriers might mean for their long-term, or not so long-term, future.

As I mentioned earlier, I can trace much of my life through a series of firsts. Many of these firsts are things everyone goes through—first day of school, first kiss, first job, first funeral or wedding attended. However, each person with CF goes through a whole series of firsts that are often unique to them.

I remember the first time I realized my body differed from other people because of the large scar gashed across my stomach. I remember the first time I saw my parents shift uncomfortably because of a question I had about the seriousness of my health. I remember the first time I understood I wouldn't be able to have kids, the first time I realized the increased coughing I was experiencing wasn't because of a long-lasting cold but because of the chronic accumulation of mucus in my lungs, the first time I was admitted to hospital, and my first intravenous line. I remember the first time I realized how scared my parents were for me. I remember the first time I learned I was not supposed to live a long life, the first time I realized I was getting sicker and I was not going to get better. And I remember the first time I cried out in the middle of the night because I thought I was choking to death on my own mucus.

So how did my mental and emotional journey into CF self-awareness begin? Well, it began of all places at the top of a waterslide and involved an unaware child and a somewhat nosy lifeguard.

In the late 1980s, a neighboring city got its first wave pool. These pools were all the rage back in the day, and like many other kids born in the 1980s, I spent many birthday parties there. The first time I went to the wave pool was with my cousin and his dad. My favorite part of any aquatic complex was the waterslides—if they didn't have waterslides, what was the point of even going?

During that inaugural trip to the wave pool, my cousin and I were zipping up and down the slides. On one of our trips up the many platforms and steps, while waiting at the mouth of the slide, the lifeguard took a second look at me and asked, "What is that scar from on your stomach?" (You may remember that earlier

I mentioned that when I was three days old, I had a surgery to remove a blockage in my bowel. Well, since then, the scar has grown with me, turning my stomach into quite a scene). I glanced at the lifeguard, a little taken aback that she would say anything more to me than the words "wait" or "go." I distinctly remember thinking, *What is a scar, and where is it on my stomach?* To me, my stomach always looked normal. There was my little pot belly, then right underneath that was the long nasty line cutting horizontally across my stomach, and then my half-inny/half-outy belly button. Nothing unusual to see here.

I turned my head towards her, a little perplexed. "What do you mean?"

"That scar across your stomach, what is it from, a surgery?"

"I . . . I don't know. It looks the same to me as it always has." I grew more and more self-conscious as kids often do when pointed out in a crowd. I hated being asked questions I didn't know the answer to, especially when it had to do with my body, and now everyone in line was checking me out. On top of all that, this teenage lifeguard was looking at me with less of a questioning look on her face and more of a look that seemed to communicate, "Are you stupid? Look at your stomach, dumbass!"

As the seconds ticked by, I felt smaller and smaller under the inquisitive and confused eyes of everyone around me. My face grew hot and I wanted to disappear. Luckily for me, the mouth of the giant waterslide was open, and I figured, *To hell with this. I'm out of here!*

I don't remember what I was thinking about on the ride down the slide, but I remember that when I got to the bottom, I stayed low in the water of the landing pool, slinking my way out of the water, purposefully keeping my eyes away from the top of the tower where I could only image the lifeguard watching this weird

Big Breath In

little kid, with a massive scar across his belly, walking in the opposite direction of her.

I made my way to the big pool, got into the waves, and, with no one watching, stole a look down at my stomach. *What is wrong with it?* I wondered. It was then that I had an idea. *This is the perfect place to compare my belly to other people's bellies.* I lifted my eyes from the water and up to the other kids and parents walking around on the deck of the pool. What met my eyes was like something I had never seen before. Everyone walking around the pool all had smooth bellies! Sure, some were bigger than others, some more round and some more flat, but they were all smooth. They didn't have the grotesque skin fold I had. Everyone just had a button-sized mark on their stomach and nothing else! *How could this be? Isn't a person's stomach supposed to have a crevice across the bottom of it? What is going on? Am I the only person with a normal-looking stomach?* I got out of the water and, for the first time in my life, instinctively held my arm at a ninety-degree angle in front of my stomach, covering my scar. As I continued to look around, it finally dawned on me: other people weren't the ones who were different; *I was the different one!*

Now, this wasn't the only time my slow-wittedness was on display, but this was the most painfully unique time in my childhood. After my mom came and picked me up, I asked her if there was something different about my stomach. Did I have that thing that the lifeguard said I had—a scar? My mom smiled and chuckled a little. I guess she always thought her son was brighter than he actually was and had instinctively put two-and-two together—after all, this wasn't the first time I had seen people in bathing suits. But sure enough, she lifted her shirt above her stomach and revealed that her stomach differed from mine also!

Over the next couple of days, I came to see that my dad's stomach was different, my brother's stomach was different, and my sister's stomach was different. Even the boys in my grade, when we went to change for PE class—all different. By now, I was understanding that there was something unique about me.

I was a boy who loved to play and have fun. Looking at other people's stomachs or appearances wasn't something I did before that waterslide incident, and I am happy about that. It meant that CF was not affecting my life much at all and that I was a happy and healthy kid. My mom retold me the story that when I was very small, I needed to have surgery to save my life. That surgery had to do with why I took pills every time I ate, why I did chest physio every day, and why we went to the hospital to talk to the doctors every three months. This wasn't the first time she told me this story, but it was the first time it sunk in. Things began falling into place. There *was* something different about me, but instead of being ashamed, I was actually kind of proud of it.

I decided I would not be ashamed of my body, but instead, I was going to flaunt it. The following September, when school started up again, I decided to show my stomach off for show-and-tell. I was, of course, super dramatic when I lifted my shirt and told my classmates about my scar and the life-saving surgery I got when I was only three days old. The class was mesmerized by the tale of my brush with death, and it felt good. That is, of course, until my best friend Garrit got it in his head to tell the story of how when he was born, he turned blue right away because the cord was wrapped around his neck and he would have definitely died even quicker than me if the doctors hadn't done something. (Come on, Garrit!)

At that same time, I also began taking pride in my pills because they also set me apart. I relished the idea that I got to skip school every three months to talk with adults, or at least listen to my mom talk to them at my CF clinic. As I would find out later in life, one of my parents' fears was that, like Warren, I would be seen as different from my peers, but at this stage in life when my *differentness* came with no consequences that prevented me from doing what I wanted to do, I was enjoying the attention (Wow, a therapist could pick this apart. #textbookattentionseeker). Unfortunately, I would not remain in this state of blissful uniqueness forever, for as I grew, I would later discover the full consequence of my differences, and when that time came, I found myself pleading to not be different anymore.

Like my first realization of differentness, perched on the top of a waterslide, this next experience of paralyzing self-awareness also came in the summer, but this time, I was alone and it was roughly seven years later. If my first real experience of differentness because of CF brought a sense of pride, then this second moment of awareness brought nothing but fear and anxiety. It was the experience of uncovering the truth that just as my stomach looked different from everyone else's, so too did my life expectancy.

By the time I turned thirteen, I worked on our dairy farm during the summer and after school, doing chores around the farm and some fieldwork on some of our smaller tractors. On one particular sunny afternoon in early August, between Grades 7 and 8, we were baling hay in one of our fields. It was after lunch, and I was supposed to head out to the field with a tractor to do some work that would help get the hay ready to be baled.

Before heading out, however, I had an hour to kill as we were waiting for the grass to dry a bit more. As my dad, mom, and sister left the yard after lunch to do the work they needed to do, I stayed inside the house and went over to our brand-new computer to play my computer games for a bit. My older sister, Lynette, was starting nursing school in the coming fall, so my parents figured it was finally time to upgrade our computer from 1987.

With this new computer, we also got the most cutting-edge computer program: *Encarta 95*. For those who are a couple of years younger than me, you may never have heard of *Encarta 95*, as the Internet soon replaced this tool. Basically put, *Encarta* was the digitalization of the encyclopedia. That's right, I said "encyclopedia."

After spending some time that afternoon playing my regular computer games, I decided to look up a couple of things on *Encarta*. For some reason, looking up topics on a computer program was much more fun than looking them up in the old encyclopedia set on the shelf. What made me type "cystic fibrosis" into the search bar I don't know, but what it said, within the first couple lines, has stayed lodged in my mind ever since: *The average life expectancy of someone with cystic fibrosis is eighteen years old.*

It felt like someone had kicked me in the stomach. I felt short of breath, even though my lung function was perfectly normal for a kid my age. I got sweaty. *Is this true? Do I only have about five years left to live?*

Now, if *Encarta* had been up to date on the latest CF research, they would have known these stats were out of date. Nonetheless, even if the life expectancy was ten years more than written, I couldn't help but be shocked at this startling revelation. Was this difference in me actually going to kill me and so soon? I began panicking. *Will I never get married? Will I never have kids? Will I never have sex?!?!* (This last question was probably the most disturbing for me being a thirteen-year-old boy). I protested. *This cannot be! I feel fine. I just finished playing ice hockey at a high level for kids my age. I am healthy. Sure, I cough a bit and take some pills, but is all this going to kill me before I even graduate high school?*

I didn't know what was going on anymore. How serious was this disease? All I knew is that I needed to get away from the computer as fast as possible! I quickly erased the search history, feeling somehow ashamed that I had read this information. For some reason, I thought that the only thing worse than me knowing this information was my parents knowing that I knew it. I ran downstairs to the back door of the house, slipped into my shoes, and ran out the door.

The hot August sun hit me with a warmth that was completely counter to the coldness I was feeling inside. Though it was still a bit early to head out to the field to begin work, I didn't care. I jumped on the tractor, but before tearing out of the yard, I noticed I needed fuel. I pulled up to the fuel tanks and began refueling, turning over in my head the information that threatened to spin me out of control. And then the seriousness of this thing hit me: *CF is going to kill me!*

My stomach churned and my lunch wanted to exit the same way it had gone in. Trying to compose myself, I began taking in deep breaths, to bring myself back to reality through the smells of the diesel fuel I was pumping into the tractor and the freshly cut grass that was drying in the next field over. I started talking myself down: *George, it's going to be okay. You are totally healthy. Look at yourself. You can run and ride your bike as fast as any of your friends. You're a star hockey player, and this year, you are even leaving your goalie net behind and playing defense, skating with the other guys! You can work like a mule. You are healthy. This stuff you just read applies to those who are really sick with CF, not you. You are going to be fine!*

I would use this same technique of breathing combined with my own personal pep talk many times over the next ten years to tell myself everything was going to be okay and that I would beat the odds. CF affects all of its victims in different ways. I told myself that I would be one of the lucky ones.

And the truth is, I *was* one of the lucky ones—uncharacteristically healthy for someone with CF, and I made sure to confirm this with my doctor during my next clinic visit. However, in all this thinking, one thing crystalized in my young mind. I would not tell my parents I knew I was dying.

Now, it was not like my parents had not tried to talk to me about CF before and lay out how serious this illness was. My parents put a lot of emphasis on raising us to be responsible kids, and explaining these things to us was part of that. I remember sitting on the kitchen counter after dinner when I was about ten. My mom was cleaning up dinner, and my dad was sitting on the couch watching TV. I was talking about how I was noticing more and more how CF was making me different. I was coughing more, taking pills that no one else took, and not to mention the huge scar I now recognized on my belly. After hearing this, my mom, trying to be sensitive and not make a big deal of it, but seeking to convey some truth to me, mentioned that because of CF, when I got older, I might get sick, need to spend time in hospital, and I would mostly likely not be able to have children of my own. However, to my later detriment, what she told me did not register in my mind with the weight it should have. What registered was the pain I saw in her eyes as she told me this. When I looked over at my dad, I also saw pain and sadness evident on his face as he listened in on the conversation. At this point, it had not been more than a year and a half since Warren had passed away. The pain and grief of his passing, though healing a little, was still very raw and tangible. I had seen the pain and grief that my parents had gone through with Warren's death, and though they had masked it well in front of my sister and me, I still knew what it looked like in their eyes—eyes of grief and sorrow never lie.

Seeing this pain creep across my parents' faces as they tried to talk to me about my health, feeling that now-familiar mood of discomfort blow into the kitchen, and not wanting to return to any of that, I simply shrugged, told them I already knew all that (an obvious lie to get out of an uncomfortable situation), and went upstairs to my room to play with my farm toys. The information they told me did not fully register, but the pain it was causing them to do so did.

Already, at this young age, I knew the reality and finality of death. I had kissed my brother's cold forehead, I had seen him lying in his casket, and I saw that casket placed over his wide-open grave. I went to his graveside with my parents and sister each birthday, Christmas, and times in-between. I had seen and lived with our grieving home, and I was not yet ready to broach this again, especially if my health would cause this. And so, at that young age, I shut it out—all I wanted to do was get as far from those feelings as possible.

I admire my parents so much for even being able to care for me during those times. How they could come home from Warren's funeral or from the numerous visits to his grave, and then do percussion physio on me and divide up the pills for me to take, constant reminders that they had *two* unhealthy sons who *both* had fatal illnesses. How they did this, what strength they had, is beyond what I can fathom, even now as an adult.

So, on that hot August afternoon, standing there refueling the tractor and letting the full impact of CF finally hit me, I decided this was going to be *my* battle and I was going to live. My parents were not going to be burying another son.

Though I decided to distract myself to get my mind off the fact that CF wanted to kill me, this reality lingered in my mind. But every time I went to those fatal thoughts, I busied myself with some sort of distraction. It was not so much a denial, but a battle against letting it consume me. I know that deciding to handle it on my own was not the healthiest thing to do. I had a loving family who wanted to help me carry this burden, but in my youthful mind I also wanted to protect them from the pain of my new-found self-awareness.

This first mental battle with CF shaped and strengthened my mental and emotional resolve, something I would need often when my health nosedived over a decade later. CF can sometimes be as much a mental battle as a physical one. When things slide, it is not only one's physical body that needs to fight, but one's mental health as well. Later, in my mid-twenties, when the bad news poured down on me in torrents and I realized that the information I had stumbled upon back in the summer of '95 was actually not that far off from my reality, I would have to fight to keep my head above water, to keep my focus and will to fight to the very end.

In some ways, young people with CF are often known to be quite mature for their age. Part of this, I believe, is due to these early mental battles, the childhood decisions, and drive to overcome the scientific odds that tell you there is very little hope of a long and healthy life.

But if reading about the outcomes of CF was one mental hurdle to leap, witnessing it in the life of another person was something very different.

Erin

Often, when I share my story, after telling about my oblivious nature on full display at the wave pool, I always say, "If, as a child, I was oblivious to the effects of CF, then my cousin Erin, who also had CF, was anything but. I am sure there was not a day in her life when she could be oblivious to the effects of CF."

Erin was an energetic girl who grew up into a young woman with a passion for life. Whether it was biking, going to Hawaii, or knee boarding while boating with her family, she wanted to be in on the action!

Erin was petite. I remember being in Grade 4 and our family pulling out of my uncle and aunt's driveway after an afternoon of visiting with them and asking how old Erin was. Hearing my mom's reply that she was only a year younger than I was astonishing, as Erin was so much shorter than me and most girls in my grade.

Erin and I were not especially close during our first twelve years. When the family got together, I played with my male cousins, and Erin played with the female cousins. But I knew that Erin and I had the unique bond of CF.

Now, what are the odds of cousins having CF? Well, usually not that high. It is a lot more common for siblings to have it, but in a totally healthy and socially acceptable way, we are somewhat close to being siblings—at least in lineage.

When my dad was young, his family lived only a seven-minute drive from my mom's family in a rural community. Both of them come from, in today's standards, somewhat larger families: my mom has five siblings and my dad has three. My parents and their siblings went to the same elementary and high schools, the same church, and most of the same social gatherings; therefore, it is not a stretch that my parents weren't the only ones from their respective families to fall in love. A couple of years after my parents were married, my mom's younger brother married my dad's younger sister; hence, the genetic cocktail known as Keulen/Luymes was once again in play, and the unknown, but fatal, one-in-four chance of a child being born with CF was again very much present. A little over eighteen months after I was born, my uncle and aunt had their second child, Erin, and she too was born with CF.

Though our genetics were similar, our experience with CF couldn't have been further apart. My first admission to hospital was not until I was fifteen. Erin, on the other hand, spent a portion of every year of her life, apart from one 365-plus-day period, in the hospital. Erin knew what it was to *suffer* from CF. She knew what it was to miss weeks of school because of the infections that CF caused in her young lungs; and she knew as a child what it was to be completely out of breath upon exertion. She also knew what it was to watch her oblivious cousin cruise through life as if he didn't even have CF, often leaving her behind in their teen years, failing to pick up on the clues that she was looking for another person with CF to talk to. But that guy was an ass, unable at the time to put himself in someone else's shoes, even someone he was supposed to love.

By the time Erin became a senior in high school, her life had become quite restricted. No more biking around their family dairy farm, other than riding on the second-seat of a tandem bike. No manual labor on the farm, although she found a job at an ice-cream shop, which she loved, until she had to quit because it too became too much for her body to handle. She knew what it was to have to leave university because of repeated hospitalizations and the inability to walk comfortably from building to building without becoming out of breath.

There were times when Erin and I were in high school and she would end up in hospital in quite serious condition, waiting for the antibiotics to kick in, not knowing which way things were going to go. I would, of course, know she was in hospital and that it was not going well, this being emphasized by how quiet our house would get. During some of those times, I would be upstairs in my room after dinner, listening to music and finishing some homework, when my dad would knock on my door and stand in the doorway. Having spoken with his sister, Erin's mom, he would tell me that things didn't look good with Erin. He would be silent for a moment and then explain how though he couldn't imagine what I was going through and what might be going through my head in watching Erin suffer as she did; he would say how sorry he was, both for Erin and for me in our separate but connected challenges, with tears often welling up in his eyes. He never wanted me to have to go through this, and though he wanted nothing more than to fix it, to protect me from this, he knew he couldn't.

During the two or three times this happened, the pain I suspected my parents carried because of CF was confirmed; not only pain but also guilt for having passed this illness on to me.

About a couple of years after Erin passed away, my parents, sister, and I were having dinner, and we somehow got onto the topic of CF and SMA. At some point in the conversation, my parents broke down, saying how sorry they were for passing these illnesses to Warren and me, saying how parents are supposed to give good things to their children, not impossible burdens. A thought germinated in my mind then, that over a decade and a half later, I would become fully convinced of: *It is often easier to suffer yourself than to watch someone you love suffer, knowing there is nothing you can do to save them.*

CF made its final assault on Erin's body in the winter of 2003, when she was only nineteen years old. Erin was admitted to hospital in early February, and on Valentine's Day, woke up knowing something was very wrong. Within an hour of waking up and calling her mom, she was rushed down to the ICU and placed in a coma so that she could be intubated. Her unconscious body waged war against the infections immanently threatening her life. She was brought out of the coma after two weeks, and though she could not come off the ventilator, she rebounded to the point of being able to walk up and down the hallways of the ICU, charming everyone in her path. However, on March 19, she once again took a turn for the worse, and the following day, CF took her young life.

For me, it was a time of disorientation. I was grieving for Erin, trying to be strong for my family, but all the while feeling guilty for what felt like my self-centeredness in wondering when this fate was going to come for me.

I felt like an elephant in the room, a constant reminder of CF's terribleness, but also a reminder of how unfair it was that here I stood, seemingly untouched by the disease, and there lay Erin, a young and passion-filled woman, now gone.

Sitting at Erin's funeral was one of the loneliest experiences of my young life, and it might also have been the most shameful. As I sat on the wooden pew near the front of a packed church, with all my family around me, all of us listening to Erin being eulogized and the pastor sharing about Erin's love for life and faith, all I could think about was myself. Every time the pastor mentioned CF, I wondered if all eyes were staring at me because that is what it felt like. Of course, no eyes were looking at me. Everyone in that church was rightfully overcome with the grief of Erin's passing, and yet I felt like there was a spotlight on me, the *other one* with CF. All I could think about was when would this fate, this funeral, these tears, be for me?

At this point, I was finishing up my second year of university, and I knew my health was slipping. I was coughing more, and I too was having more trouble walking from building to building on campus. I knew that the fault lines of my own health were growing ever wider.

As I look back now, though I was still holding my own—healthy enough to play on the university hockey team and work for several years on our dairy farm—2003 was one of the most difficult years of my life. I look back and hardly recognize my memories of that year. More so than the years when my own life was becoming smaller and smaller because of CF, when I found myself unable to breathe, no longer able to work, and spending more and more time in hospital. It was that year—the year of watching Erin's life slip away, seeing the raw marks of grief on the faces of people I loved, living through the real-life reminder of just how fragile life with CF is—it felt all too much.

It is clear to see how transitional that year was for the rest of my life. Looking back, it is easy to see that without knowing it, CF was already taking over center stage in my life. My carefree days were disappearing. CF had taken Erin's life, and it was clear, without even realizing it at the time, it was now coming for me. I was dealing with all the regular things someone in their early twenties deals with, but now doing so through the ever-thickening lens of cystic fibrosis.

4.
TYPICAL 20S (WITH A CF LENS)

> "We may spend our whole life climbing the ladder of success, only to find when we get to the top our ladder is leaning against the wrong building."
>
> (*Falling Upward,* Richard Rohr)

WHEN ERIN PASSED away, CF had already become a fixture in my life. Though I was still quite healthy and could participate in most activities, CF had its grip on me. Back in my senior year of high school, I could feel CF's effects slowly creeping up. After running in PE class or playing ice hockey, it would always take me a couple minutes to catch my breath and get my coughing under control. I could tell that people were also noticing my worsening symptoms.

After graduating high school in 2000, I took a year off from school and worked on our family dairy farm. I always loved working on the farm. The cows were not my first vocational choice, but tell me to spend the day on the tractor working out in the field and I would be in my sweet spot. I loved tractors and heavy machinery. Ever since I can remember, I have loved to drive—from those early days trying out Warren's wheelchair to driving the farm truck around the yard and laneways when I was eight. I admit I wasn't very good at negotiating corners at that young age, something that can be hard to do when you can barely see over the steering wheel, so sure enough, I sideswiped the garage on an occasion or two. But I loved being behind the wheel. During this gap year, I also developed a second love. Okay, "love" might be the wrong word here. It was more of an addiction—running!

Now that I was spending a lot of time sitting in a tractor, I wanted to become more intentional in my activity level, so I took up running. I never minded running, and I have always enjoyed pushing myself. Running, like so many other endurance activities, is not really all that *fun* when doing it, although it can be on those days when you feel full of energy. But it is one of those things that makes you feel amazing afterwards. After each run, I would look down at my wristwatch and see that I had run for thirty or forty-five minutes and be filled with a sense of satisfaction. Of course, I could only get a quick glance at my watch before I would be bent over coughing up all the mucus that had come loose during the run. After my airways cleared and I was once again taking in big comfortable breaths, it was as if I were standing on a mountain vista. Overall, I took good care of myself that first year after high school. But I soon found myself wanting to go back to school.

While a senior in high school, and during the year that I spent on the farm, faith and spiritually, which had been part of my life growing up, started becoming more and more important to me. Reflecting on the circumstances of my struggle with CF, Warren's death, and all the other suffering I saw going on around me, I began feeling that there had to be more to this life than what I could simply see and touch. All the suffering happening around me had to mean something. I know many people see the world's suffering and become turned off by the idea of a God, and I understand that. For me, that was not so much the issue, and in fact, I still struggle with the idea of suffering, meaning, and the question of *why*. But it was more that I could not believe that life—that Warren's life and death, Erin's suffering, and my own CF—were just a random series of biological events strung together to create a life that, in the end, would be suffocated out of existence with no further recourse or meaning. I couldn't seem to abide by a worldview where there is nothing more—where we simply live the life we have by chance, try to be respectful citizens for the common good, and then die. There had to be something outside of my own existence and reality to find hope, meaning and value in. And I found that meaning and value in the Judeo-Christian faith—a spirituality based in love, grace, hope, and peace.

As my faith became more important in my life, I decided to transition out of farming and back to school. In the fall of 2001, I enrolled at a local University, intending to become a pastor. This was a four-year bachelor of arts that would then pave the way to get my master's degree.

The Danger of 20-Something

In the CF community, everyone knows that one's early twenties are a critical time for CF patients (this is also the case in other illness too). Though one is emerging into adulthood, one often still acts like an adolescent. This phase of life, considering yourself an adult but still harboring some immature attitudes and lack of awareness, can often spell disaster for someone suffering with serious health challenges. If a person with CF can stay healthy through their early to mid-twenties, then the future is often very bright for them. CFers often take a huge hit to their health during this chapter of life, however, and I was no exception.

My first year of university went by just fine. Knowing that I could no longer go for my summer runs, my parents bought a treadmill, and most mornings before class, I would go for a thirty-minute run on it in the garage. I really enjoyed that first year and made it through almost unscathed from any further effects from CF. Then my sister and some friends decided they wanted to hike the West Coast Trail. The West Coast Trail is a five-to-seven-day hike. It runs along the western-most part of Vancouver Island, on the west coast of Canada. It is a grueling hike through coastal forest trails filled with mud, stretches where you have to walk over long sandy beaches, climb up and down wooden ladders full of slippery moss, pull yourself over rivers by rickety old cable cars, and of course, pack in and out all of your supplies for the whole week you are out there in the Canadian coastal wilderness.

Until this time, I had been doing a lot of running, and encouraged by my sister, I decided the hike would be a good challenge and accomplishment to have under my belt. It turned out to be more challenging than fun, but an amazing experience it was. A couple members of our group wanted to push the pace, so we went a bit faster than I would have liked, but I did it. Each morning, we rolled out of our cold tents into the moist ocean air. Most nights, we set up our tents right on the beach of the Pacific Ocean, where all you could hear was the constant crashing of waves. The first thing I would do in the morning would be to take a couple puffs of Ventolin and begin using my PEP mask to help move some of the mucus out of my lungs in order to give myself a bit of an advantage once we got hiking. Throughout the day, I would take a couple more hits from my puffer when I needed it, but with all the challenging terrain that we hiked over, I didn't need to do much extra physio. I am incredibly proud that I have done this hike. We finished the hike in five days, one day ahead schedule. But the trip also marked a negative turning point in my life, one that often overshadows the experience of the hike.

I point to hiking the West Coast Trail as the last thing I did before I got sick. It marks the last time that I would consider myself to be carefree and healthy. After coming back from the hike, it was like my body was telling me, *Okay, we did that, you've had your fun. Now it is time for CF to have its turn.* It was in the weeks and months following the hike that CF placed a firmer grip on my life, a grip that would never let go.

For some reason, after the hike, I stopped running. I was not the most serious runner, but at least four or five times a week, I would be on the treadmill in the morning or outside on the local sea wall in the evening. But after the West Coast Trail, I never picked up running again. Instead, "life" took over. Things got more and more busy. If I was not in class or studying, I was helping in a drama club I had joined. If I was not doing that, I was helping in my church youth group. And if I was not doing any of those things, on the weekends, I would be found working on the farm and hanging out with friends. I was losing myself in my life, and I was not paying attention to the effects this new busyness was having on my health. When I found the motivation to go to the gym or for a run, I no longer had the energy to do it because I was not allowing the proper downtime for my body to rest. I was still doing my physio twice a day and taking all my pills, but as a CF patient, I was also committing the most unforgivable sin—I was minimizing and ignoring the increasing symptoms of CF. This was my state as I entered 2003 and everything that year brought with it.

This is why one's early twenties can be so detrimental for people with CF. People in their twenties often think they are invincible, that things will just work out, and that the worst will never happen. I refused to listen to advice and just wanted to do things my way, to live the way I always had. Everyone else was living busy lives, why couldn't I?

I was not spending my time drinking and partying as many people do in this stage of life, but I may as well have been—at least I might have gotten more sleep. Instead, I was grinding myself thin with a full schedule and ignoring the ever-increasing symptoms of CF. The more tired and weaker I got, the stronger and more dominant CF became. The balance of power was shifting.

Erin passed away near the end of my second year of university. Now, one would think that if I had any sort of sense, this would have been a wake-up call to get my health back on track and start taking better care of myself. But it wasn't. I had become so good at minimizing and ignoring my symptoms, or explaining away any weakness or deterioration in my health, that I wasn't allowing myself to see it any other way.

Why can I no longer run 30 minutes but instead only 15 minutes? It's no big deal. It's just because I haven't been training.

Why am I coughing so much just from walking across campus? Well, I do have CF. What do you expect?

Why do I wake up twice a night to cough when I've never had to do this before? Well . . . uh . . . well, I still get enough sleep. I'm sure it'll go away.

The excuses were there when I needed them, and if they didn't work, I simply ignored the ever-increasing fatal symptoms. My doctors saw things were slipping. They looked at me with a critical eye and told me I needed to slow down. Hospitalization started coming up more and more in conversation, but I was mostly able to keep them off my back. I downplayed how out of breath I really got. I did not do this deceptively; I just truly believed that I was as healthy as I was telling them. I was not lying to *them*, but I was lying to *myself*. An accurate picture of my health was not being seen. X-rays and pulmonary function tests can only go so far in painting the picture of someone's health. Everyone is different, and without the patient's honesty and participation in their care, there is only so much the doctors can do. Therefore, the true reality of my declining health went unnoticed, both by me, and because of that, my doctors.

My greatest fear at this time was hospitalization. I was very familiar with hospitals. Being in them did not freak me out, but being admitted was another story. In my mind, only sick people are admitted to hospitals. I saw Erin grow up in and out of hospitals. *I am not Erin*, I told myself. I saw my brother die in the hospital. I was not going to die. I was one of the healthy ones! With each passing clinic visit, it became my goal to keep myself out of the hospital. Other than a quick procedure in the tenth grade, I had never been hospitalized, and to pass over that threshold from being an out-patient to an in-patient meant that I was now admitting that I was *sick*. I kept telling myself that I was not sick, just a little rundown. I mean, just look at me, *cough, cough, wheeze, wheeze*.

I often wonder how many more years I could have gotten out of my lungs if I had paid more attention to my doctors' advice and my parents' warnings to slow down. If I had been more open to being hospitalized for the sake of maintenance and prevention, would I still be breathing with my original lungs? If I had taken the concern on my parents' faces more seriously, could I have saved them years of premature stress and anguish as they watched their second son dying in front of their eyes?

In my early 20s, there was still time to turn the ship around. I was not growing any serious bacteria. Things could easily have been controlled if I had just woken up and smelled the coffee—or smelled the infections. But I was living life in the fast lane—getting grades I never thought possible (I was never much of a student until university), being a mentor to a group of guys, learning and displaying leadership skills I never knew I had, and receiving accolades and recognition along the way. Why would I slow down? I told myself, *If I was doing all these things then I must be healthy.*

I had this idea that if I started out at a certain level of healthiness, it would take me that much longer to get sick than those who had always been sicker than me. I reasoned that if I could still function at this level, it would take another fifteen years to get really sick, and by that time, I would be done school, I would have settled down, and then my health would obviously bounce back. So, I kept going, convincing myself I was healthy and denying the truth that I was busying myself to death.

Catching a Breather and Changing Course

My third year of university continued much like the second. I had taken on a larger leadership role in the youth program of my church, so if I was not at school or studying, I was working at the church, planning activities and discussions. This kind of schedule put any intentions of exercise to rest. Exercise is such an important part of CF treatment, which had been proven in my life just a couple of years earlier. But with life getting in the way, I turned my back on my exercise regimen and, as far as I can remember, never went for a real run again.

However, there came a glimmer of hope in my fourth year. In preparing for graduation, and with the possibility of doing graduate work on the horizon, I took a heavy course load, which forced me to step down from my position in church and focus only on school. To paint a picture of my health at this time, I could still walk wherever I needed to go but had bouts of coughing and shortness of breath upon arrival at my destination. Early morning classes were a little embarrassing, as the first couple minutes of the professor's lectures would be punctuated by my coughing, the residual mucus still making its way out of my lungs from my morning physio. I was finally becoming self-conscious about my coughing. Each morning, I would drive onto campus, park my car, and then wait until I could not see anyone else in the parking lot. I would then get out of my car, take two big breaths of air, heave my backpack over my shoulders, and begin walking towards the lecture halls. I would try to make sure I was out of earshot of other commuters, for as soon as the cold air hit my airways, I was thrown into a coughing fit that would last one to two minutes.

However, during my final year of university, I began noticing small improvements in my health. I was able to find more time to work out now that my schedule was not stretched so thin. Since anytime I tried running I would just end up in a coughing-out-of-breath fit after just forty-five seconds, I began working out with weights. I was putting on more weight and feeling more comfortable than I ever had over the previous two years. As graduation approached and final papers were handed in, things were looking up, as I always told myself they would. But I had a decision to make: Would I continue on in school, apply for a master's program, and pursue a career as a pastor, or would I chalk up my four years of university to a great experience and training for future volunteer work, and head back to the farm to pursue a career alongside my dad? When it came right down to it, the decision was quite easy to make.

During my final semester, the weather was horrible. Really, this was no surprise. The west coast of Canada is not called the "Wet Coast" for nothing. It was around mid-February, and we were in the middle of a full month of dreary rain. I was researching for a paper on the third floor of the university library. It was mid-afternoon, but the weather was so dark that it almost looked like

Big Breath In

it was already evening. As I sat, trying to study, bored out of my mind, I peered out the window to the ground below, to the back of the cafeteria and the university's garbage collection area. In the driving rain, a groundskeeper was out in full rain gear, collecting garbage and filling a dumpster. At that moment, as I sat in the warm, comfortable library, a realization hit me: I envied that guy out there!

Now, of course, I didn't envy him because of the work he was doing—I never really had any aspirations of becoming a groundskeeper—but I envied him because he was outside working with his hands, even if it was in the cold rain. And more importantly, he wasn't in a library researching for an academic paper he really didn't care about. I figured, *Why spend years doing work that I don't enjoy when I would rather be doing something outside with my hands?* My decision was made. I was done with school. Over the previous four years, I had seen my health deteriorate from being able to run forty-five minutes to barely being able to walk up a flight of stairs without coughing. It was time to get back to my roots. I was a farmer. Was my faith still important to me? Absolutely. But the farm was where I belonged—working the land, taking care of animals, breathing in the outside fresh air, and being more physical than I had been in years. That was where I wanted to be.

And so, the day after donning my cap and gown, I was up at 5:00 a.m., beginning what I thought would be a long and healthy career as a dairy farmer.

5.
BREAK DOWN

> "When we have been prevented
> from learning how to say no,
> our bodies may end up saying it for us."
>
> (*When the Body Says No,* Gabor Mate, MD)

AFTER GRADUATING UNIVERSITY, I hit the ground running. Working on the farm and being outside again felt great. Building up calluses on my hands, taking on more responsibility, and feeling the freedom of being an adult all made for a great work experience.

Within a couple of months of graduation, I moved into my own place. This was a house that my parents owned on one of their farm properties. We fixed it up over the summer, and in early September, I moved in. I decorated the place myself and made it my own. Of course, I was only twenty-three years old, so to the outside eye, it was rather bare, with the regular cluttered countertop of a bachelor pad—dishes in the sink, dust and dirt collecting around the floorboards and on most surfaces—but it was *my* place.

My work schedule was pretty standard for dairy farming: up at 5:00 a.m. each day, a break for breakfast and lunch, and done work around 6:00 p.m. I got every second weekend off. Farming was and still is my first vocational passion. But this season of life not only brought a change in vocation and housing, but it also brought a change to my relationship status.

Kim and I had known each other since the eighth grade, but we never captured each other's eye in high school; the closest we got was having a couple of mutual friends. However, after high school, a number of our friends disappeared off to out-of-town universities, and we all of a sudden found ourselves thrown into a small mix of people, hanging out most weekends. Over the following years, I dated a number of girls for various lengths of time, but they always ended in heartbreak—either theirs or mine. At the beginning of my fourth year of university, while focusing on studies and not spread so thin, the depth of friendship Kim and I had developed began to turn into something more (think Chandler and Monica ☺). Now, this wasn't the end of the story, or even the beginning. It was only the introduction, as it would still be a year before we would give dating its first short-term go, thus beginning a two-year on-and-off-again story (think Ross and Rachel). But something deep (and complicated) was taking shape.

In late 2005, now farming and living on my own, I also got my first taste of traveling, heading down to the Dominican Republic with a group of friends. This trip was a little awkward, as we booked it when Kim and I were dating, but by the time of the trip, we had broken up (part of that pesky two-year on-and-off-again story). The trip however did wonders for my health, with my lungs thriving in the warm and relaxing setting.

My health throughout 2005 was fairly good, but in 2006, it once again began to slip. At work, I had to watch it. I began wearing a mask during particularly dusty work after it seemed I had developed a kind of short-term clot in my lungs that caused a lot of chest pain. This went away after a couple of days, and I returned to normal. My parents also had a closer eye on my health because I was working on the farm and would recommend I take more time off when needed. But, like in university, this was not an offer I often took them up on.

During those two-and-a-half years after university, my alarm would go off at 5:00 a.m. Groggily, I would get dressed and drive the five minutes to the farm. I'd pop my head into the milking parlor to say, "Mornin'" to my dad and then head out to feed the cows. I would start with checking and cleaning the maternity pen, but this was also a strategic move on my part. In this pen, there was a short concrete wall, about three feet high, where I could sit.

I had now been awake for about fifteen minutes, and the mucus that had collected in my lungs overnight would be loosened up. I would make my way into the barn with the maternity pen, duck under the neck railing where the cows would eat, and sit on this low wall. I would then lean forward with my hands on my knees and purposefully begin hacking my lungs out! It usually took about three to five minutes to pull the mucus up and out of my lungs, and then another minute to catch my breath. By the time, I finished there would be about five-tablespoons of mucus at my feet that I would shovel some cow shit over. The cows in the maternity pen would just lay there looking at me, or one would hobble over, getting a better look at this poor sap making these horrendous coughing noises. Then, since she was up, she would begin sniffing around for the hay I was supposed to be feeding her. This was my cue to get moving.

From here, my workday started for real. First on my list was feeding the cows and heifers, which usually took a little more than an hour. By this time, my dad would be finished up milking, and I would begin washing the milking parlor as the last cow was leaving it. After all the milking, feeding, and washing were done, my parents and I would have breakfast at around 7:00 a.m. After a traditional farmer's breakfast of oatmeal, eggs, and toast, I would drive home, dive under the covers for a forty-five-minute nap, and then begin an hour of chest physiotherapy.

It was then back to the farm by 9:45-ish, work until 12:45-ish, and then have some lunch. After lunch, often without realizing it, I would sit with my head resting on my arms at the table. When I developed this habit, my parents often urged me to head back home and take a quick afternoon nap. I would ignore them, but if they saw I was overly run down, they would take over my afternoon work duties, thus giving me nothing to do for a couple of hours. In the summer, I often fell asleep on their couch, or in the shade of the tree-hedge behind the house.

At 3:30 p.m., afternoon milking began. I would once again feed the cows and heifers, wash down the milking parlor, and finally head home for the day. I'd make myself a quick and unhealthy processed dinner, do my thirty minutes of physiotherapy, jump in the shower, and be out the door to hang out with friends, only to wake up the following morning at 5:00 a.m. to try do it all over again.

Reading it like this, it might not sound like too busy or strenuous a schedule, and for a healthy person, it is nothing out of the ordinary—it might even be on the lighter side of manual labor. But for someone whose lung capacity was now dropping close to, if not under, 50%, this schedule began to take its toll. During this time, I felt myself getting more and more out of breath with the simple task of walking. My main goal during my CF clinic visits was to downplay my symptoms and keep out of the hospital. During one of these visits, one of my CF doctors told me I was a *minimalist*, meaning I did everything in my power to minimize my symptoms. I took some offense to this as I hadn't even realized I was doing it, but something in what she said struck a chord.

Break Down

My doctors were also becoming more concerned about my health, as it wasn't long, in the fall of 2006, that I had another clinic visit and another of my CF doctors sat me down for a conversation. It went something like this.

"George, when we look at your numbers, what we see is a steady decline. It has been going on for a couple of years already. There was a nice bump in your numbers about two-years ago (final year of university), but that has now been erased. Whereas before you were considered quite healthy for someone with CF, you are now slipping into dangerous territory. It is as if you are standing on a precipice. If you begin to take care of yourself, make some hard changes in life, you'll be able to back your way off this precipice as you have done before. But if you keep going this way, if something happens, or you catch some bad bacteria, you may very well find yourself on a slippery slope."

I heard the message he was giving me. I heard it and I respected what he was saying. I didn't want to go over that precipice, but I also didn't know what life would look like if I followed his instructions. My work was my life, and there was nothing else I wanted to do. Those who looked out for me (parents, sister, and doctors) were sounding the alarm. But I was so deep in my own disillusion I had no clue what I needed to do to pull myself back.

I got home from that clinic visit, told my parents what the doctor had said, and took the rest of the day off. I wanted to take this to heart. I wanted to get better, but within a week, I was back at work, trying to keep up with everyone else.

However, without even knowing it, it was already too late. The warning that my doctor gave, "If something happens or you catch some bad bacteria," ended up being somewhat prophetic. While I made some improvement in my time management and paid more attention to my physiotherapy, I learned three months later that *something* was already happening. At my next clinic visit, my sputum sample contained a deadly bacterium called *Pseudomonas*, an often indestructible and fatal bacteria for people with CF. Turns out, it was already nesting and reproducing in my lungs.

The Hawaii Incident (Fall 2006)

Right around this time, Kim and I were in the middle of our two-year on-again-off-again relationships. We were in an "off-again" phase, and it would stay this way until we eventually found our timing the following spring. I also found myself exhausted after a long fall harvest. I did not yet know about the new and deadly bacteria I was growing, but it was taking its toll, and I felt I needed a sun-filled vacation, a time to rest and relax. Since the previous year's trip to the Dominican had done wonders for my health, I figured that a week or two of lying on a beach in the middle of the Pacific Ocean would do the trick. The only problem was that with many of my friends getting married over the previous year, or building their own businesses, the only person who was single with disposable income was Kim. And so once again, we found ourselves somewhat awkwardly going on a warm winter vacation together, having unfortunately just broken up again.

The vacation became a trip from hell before the plane's wheels even got off the runway in Vancouver. Although I should clarify, it had nothing to do with Kim or our relationship. Though Vancouver is in Canada, we actually get very little snow, which means the main international airport is rather under-equipped when it comes to major snow events. The day we left for Hawaii, we got hit with a snowstorm. We got away from the terminal okay but had to wait about thirty minutes to be de-iced and then taxi out to the runway. As we got to the edge of the runway, the pilots going through their final checklists, it appeared something was off. As passengers, we could tell it was taking longer than usual to get set on the runway. The engines would rev up, then down. After about five minutes, the captain came on the intercom to tell us a warning light had come on, and we were heading back to the terminal to get a mechanic to check it out. We taxied back to the terminal and waited in the airplane for two hours. The mechanic came on board, checked everything out, and found that the warning light was faulty. The cabin was then closed back up, and we were once again pushed away from the terminal. However, it had now been snowing all day, and the lineup for de-icing was over an hour long. It was three hours after our scheduled take-off time that we finally got off the ground, and we still had to fly the five and a half hours to our Hawaiian destination.

With all this time in the airplane, breathing in the recycled air, I began fading fast. My lungs were chock-full of mucus, and I was having problems with the cabin air pressure, which caused me to panic a bit. Once we landed, I staggered to get my bags, tugging them along behind me. A shuttle brought us to our hotel where Kim checked us in as I sat hunched in the lobby, trying to catch my breath. I comforted myself by thinking I just needed to do some physio, get a good night sleep, have a restful day on the beach, and then I'd be fine.

However, the following day brought no relief. I couldn't lay on the beach due to the pooling of mucus in my lungs, nor could I sleep well. I also felt uncomfortable, for though Kim and I were very close, she had never seen the extent of how sick I was. Actually, I had never seen the full extent of how sick I was.

On the third day, we went for a drive around the island, and I could hardly get out of the car. At Pearl Harbor, I sat on a bench as Kim took in all the sights (luckily, I had seen them already on a childhood trip). When we got back to the rental car agency, which was a block from our hotel, I sat on my haunches in front of the counter, waiting for the agent to finish talking on the phone as I found it difficult to stand. While walking the single city block back to our hotel, I had to stop three times. Then, I had to stop halfway through the hotel lobby and another time once we got off the elevator. That night, we did something I had never done before: we ordered room service. I couldn't even leave the room for dinner.

I phoned my sister and mom that evening to tell them what was going on. We decided that the following morning Kim and I would book flights so I could come home earlier than expected. We all knew we were dealing with something we had never dealt with before. What we had thought was a matter of being rundown was turning out to be something far more serious. The hope of a relaxing beach vacation was over, now I was just hoping to make it home. However, before that hope could become a reality, things went from bad to worse. A couple of hours after talking to my mom and sister, while laying down, I felt a kind of *pop* in my lungs. I'd felt this before, but never to this extent. I ran to the bathroom as I began coughing. I barged through the door and spat into the sink. What came out was pure blood!

Hemoptysis

Hemoptysis (the coughing up of blood from the lungs) is not an altogether rare thing for people with CF, but it also isn't a good thing. There is a scene in the movie *Moulin Rouge* (spoiler alert) in which the main character, played by Nicole Kidman, is coughing, and when she pulls her hand away from her mouth, you see she has coughed up blood. At this point, you know she is going to die by the end of the movie. In any movie, when someone coughs up blood, you know it is a death sentence. Now, this isn't true for people with CF (or anyone, for that matter), but it certainly doesn't help or do anyone any good.

I had been having bouts of hemoptysis since the fall of 2004. It was not a symptom I minimized, and my health care team knew all about it. The vast majority of bleeds had not been very serious and often resolved themselves on their own. These would usually happen after doing physio, or if my lungs were being irritated by something, such as dust or excessive coughing. Sometimes it would even happen while I was driving. The majority of the time though it wouldn't be more than a couple teaspoons of blood. However, there is one instance that was seared into my brain, as it was the first time I thought I was going to die.

About a year before the trip to Hawaii, I had recently moved into my own place and was working long hours. I went to bed feeling tired, but that was nothing out of the ordinary. However, at 4:00 a.m. I awoke, face down in my pillow, gasping for air. I turned my head to the side and began coughing. Blood and mucus poured out of my mouth, and, in that moment, a strange sensation washed over me. It was that feeling you get when your leg falls asleep, but this time it felt like my whole body had fallen asleep. I was paralyzed! I lay on my stomach, my face half smothered in my pillow, trying with all my might to cough up the pooling blood in my airways while also trying to suck oxygen in. All the while, my body felt like it weighed a thousand pounds, and I could not lift my head, arms, or legs to try and roll over. I began to cry, then whispered in desperation, "Help me, God. Save me. Help me, God. Save me." I didn't know if I was saying these words to save me in this life or whatever awaited me in the next, but I knew I was in trouble. After about thirty seconds of coughing, gagging, and struggling to get the accumulated fluids out of my airways, I felt a tingling sensation in my arms and legs. As I coughed, spat, and drooled onto my pillow, I began regaining some feeling in my arms and legs, slowly dragging them back and forth over the top of my mattress like a starfish. As the feeling and strength in my extremities slowly returned, I right away felt a warm sensation in my midsection and instinctively knew I had lost control of my bladder. I had no ability to stop it. After about a minute of moving my arms and legs, now lying in my urine, I finally rolled myself over onto my side, off the bed, and onto the floor. I crawled to the bathroom, sat on the toilet, grabbed a bucket from under the sink, and tried to cough up anything left in my lungs. For the most part, though, it had all ended up in my bed and pillow.

I stripped down, stumbled around to find my Ventolin puffer, took a number of hits, and then once again sat down to cough up anything more that I could. By this point, my strength had returned, and I could walk fine, but I found myself very sore and weak. I had a shower, stripped my bed, and struggled to throw everything into the washing machine. I drove to the farm, told my dad I would not be able to work, went and woke up my mom, and told her what had happened. I then fell asleep on their couch, too scared to try sleeping again in my own house.

I went to the CF clinic the following day, but the doctors had no answers for me. They had never heard of paralysis caused by hemoptysis. Their best guess was that the bleeding cut off my oxygen supply long enough that I blacked out, but came to when I instinctively began choking and coughing out some of the blood. Whatever it was, I was terrified for days to fall asleep. That was the first time I had been frightened to the core of my being, but I was lucky that it resolved itself. The bleeding stopped, I regained feeling, and within a couple days, I was back to normal.

Back to the Hawaii trip from hell. As soon as I felt the *pop* in my lungs and raced to the bathroom to cough up the bright red blood into the white porcelain sink, I knew it was going to be a bad bleed. It was not so much that this was pure blood I was coughing up, but it was that as soon as I unleashed the first mouthful, I felt a torrential gurgling in my lungs. The second mouthful of blood was already charging up my trachea, ready to burst out all over that pristine bathroom sink and countertop. It was a gushing of blood I had never felt before, and it was not stopping—it felt as if I was drowning!

For the first couple of minutes of coughing, I had the door closed, but soon Kim started knocking and asking how I was. I knew this would not end well, so between coughing and gurgles, I told her how bad it was. I then opened the door and let her in. I can only imagine what she thought as her eyes took in what looked like a grisly murder scene. The faucet was running full blast, all the handles were covered in blood, and blood spattered all over the counter and halfway up the mirror.

As things slowed down a bit and I caught my breath, I told her to call the front desk and ask them to call a cab, I needed to get to the hospital. The front desk sent someone up with a wheelchair and brought me down to a waiting cab. In the meantime, I had changed my pants and put on a clean shirt.

The cab driver could see how much distress I was in and drove well over the speed limit, even running a couple of red lights. I wasn't complaining. During the ride, Kim was getting my medical services card and travel insurance in order.

When we pulled into the ER parking lot, Kim ran in to explain what was happening and to get a wheelchair for me. After sitting for a minute, I lost my patience. I got out of the cab and tried making for the door. I only ended up taking three steps before having to sit down on the nearest curb. I looked up, and there was Kim with a nurse, bringing a wheelchair to come and get me. I got into the ER. The first thing they did was put an oxygen saturation

Big Breath In

meter on my finger, which showed that my blood oxygen was only at 63%. Anything under 88% is bad! How I was even conscious, I do not know.

To be honest, I don't know what they all did to me, other than putting an oxygen mask on me, turning it on high, and pumping Ventolin into the oxygen mix. They put an intravenous (IV) line in for antibiotics, and I can only assume steroids, because within an hour, I actually started feeling pretty good. During the hour it took to get me stabilized, Kim called my sister and got her to talk with the doctor to figure out what was going on and what they were giving me. My sister called my mom, who right away called an airline and got herself a ticket for the first flight to Hawaii.

When Kim told me that my mom was flying out, I thought this was a bit ridiculous. I got a hold of my dad and told him I was "fine." I was actually feeling quite good, and it made no sense for Mom to fly out, as I was going to try to fly home first thing that following day. My dad calmed me down and told me to let Mom come see me.

It was obvious that I was in a steroid-induced state at this point because as soon as I told the doctor of my plan to fly home, she pretty much laughed in my face. What I didn't realize is that I was actually in the ICU by this point. Medically and legally, I was in absolutely no shape to fly. She said I most likely wouldn't be released from hospital for at least a week or two.

When my mom arrived at the hospital around noon the following day, I had been moved up to the third floor, but as predicted, I ended up spending nine days in the hospital in Hawaii. Kim flew home on what was our original return flight three days after I was admitted, and the hotel we were staying in allowed my mom to stay in vacant rooms at a discounted rate.

I was flown home by medical escort, needing oxygen for most of the flight and a wheelchair to get me through the Oahu and then Vancouver airports. Once we landed, I was taken straight to St. Paul's Hospital, where I spent three more days and then another two weeks on home IV antibiotics. If two months earlier I had been standing on a precipice, as my doctor had said, I had now clearly fallen off the cliff, hit a number of sharp rocks, and was now sliding down a very slippery slope with nothing to stop me. Though we didn't know it, the road to transplant had already begun.

Repairing the Lungs, Finding my Heart (I know, a very cheesy heading)

In February 2007, three months after my little trip to the Hawaiian hospital, my CF doctors broached the topic of transplant for the first time. Since Hawaii, I kept having small bouts of hemoptysis, although nothing like I'd had on the trip. In conjunction with this, I was not rebounding from the chest infection as fast as my doctors thought I would. Therefore, transplantation was something we had to begin thinking about.

The first transplant conversation was short, but the idea was broached that I should have a meet-and-greet with the transplant team for them to get to know me and me to get to know them—this is often how these first meetings go. I figured it was a sure thing, this meet-and-greet; however, it didn't materialize. Unbeknownst to me, after my clinic visit that day, my CF doctors conferred with each other and decided to give me another year to see if I could pull my health out of the gutter. Everyone, including myself, was still quite stunned by how sick I had gotten and how damaging it was. It was clear that I was now growing some nasty bacteria that was proving hard to kill, but we were still hoping that with some intentional hard work, I might be able to pull my health back to the top of the hill I'd just fallen down.

Big Breath In

As an adult, this was my first hospitalization, and until this point, I was still working full-time on the farm. In 2007, the popularity of and access to a double-lung transplant was not nearly what it is today. It is still rare today to receive such a transplant, but back in 2007, it was almost like winning a local lottery.

However, there was another pressing issue: the rather constant bleeding in my lungs and the damage it was causing my airways. What was decided at that clinic visit, and followed through very quickly, was that I would need an embolization—a cauterizing of the blood vessel in my lungs that kept rupturing and causing the bleeds.

Other than a hospitalization in Grade 10 and the debacle that was Hawaii, this was the first time I was admitted for a procedure. (Can you really call it being admitted if it's only day surgery?) I was admitted to day-surgery, which just happened to be on the same floor as the CF clinic and in-patient ward, which was still closer to being admitted than I was comfortable with at this time. The prep for the surgery went quick enough: an IV was inserted in my arm and I was told to take off all my clothes. They were going to do the embolization of the problem blood vessel in my lungs by going through my groin—threading a catheter up into the pulmonary artery, and into my left lung.

As we got going with the procedure, the doctor first had to make a small incision in my groin so he could get at the artery that came down from my lungs. They then had to keep a lot of pressure on that incision so that it didn't open up and cause me to bleed out. They inserted the catheter, watching it on a TV screen as it threaded its way up the right side of my body through an artery, slowing coming to a stop as it entered my lung.

From CT scans, X-rays, and ongoing ultrasound, they were able to find the bulge of tissue in my lung from which they assumed the bleeds were originating. They literally burned (cauterized/

embolized) the blood vessel, thus plugging it from bleeding again. At this point, I was coughing up trace amounts of blood most of the time, so the hope was that this procedure would put a stop to that. The procedure worked but not perfectly.

For a number of days after the procedure, I still had streaks of blood in my mucus, which made me nervous. The bleeding improved after the embolization, but I also had to accept the new state of my damaged lungs. I was going to have to be careful with my coughing, to cough hard enough to bring up the mucus, but not too hard to risk another bleed.

The worst part of the procedure, however, was not the procedure at all, but what had to happen after. For six hours after the procedure, I had to lie perfectly still and apply constant pressure to the insertion site. Now, one thing you should know about me is I am one of those guys who is often changing positions in his chair, tapping his foot, or drawing in a notebook. I can't sit still. As a kid in church, I was always fussing and moving around in the wooden pew. To this day, Kim often needs to lay a hand on my leg whenever we are sitting somewhere as my constant leg thumping shakes the floor around us. So, it was torture to lie perfectly still with pressure applied to my groin to ensure the incision they made would remain stitched up and not burst open.

I was on the road to recovery within a week, doing forty-five minutes of physio each morning, and then another thirty in the evening. I also began returning to work on the farm.

It was also around this time that my dad laid his cards on the table. One afternoon in early spring 2007, about four months after Hawaii, my dad and I were having lunch. I was picking up more hours again after the embolization, and we were talking about how I was feeling. He mentioned he would like to offer me a new job. The job, he said, was to take care of myself and trying to remain as healthy as possible. Basically, he was willing to pay me my regular salary to stay home and stay healthy. Of course, he didn't actually need to tell me that this was a possibility; I always knew this was how my parents felt. I had heard their warnings and encouragement to take more time off. I knew what Warren's death had done to them, and the concern they had for me. But in my stubbornness, this was not an offer I could accept. This would not make me happy and would likely send me into depression. For better or for worse, my attitude had always been "all-in or all-out." I had yet to learn that moderation is often the key to life.

I thanked my dad for the offer but told him it would bring me no joy to do what he was offering. I loved the work and would try to do it in a healthier and safer way. We decided I would begin my workday at 9:30 a.m., and that I wouldn't need to do certain kinds of work because the environment was too unhealthy. There was also a very clear understanding that at any time at all, in any situation, I could get up and walk away—to go home and do physio and rest if I needed it or quit and take up his offer to work on my health full-time.

The way I worked, however, was not the only big change that came in spring 2007. While spending some less time at work and more time at home, I became lonelier, reflecting more on my life and what was truly important.

For many people with CF, the idea of marriage, or lifelong partnership, can cause a lot of anxiety. I have spoken with people who wonder about the idea of committing to a lifelong relationship with someone they love, knowing that there is a good chance they may die young, thus leaving their partner with a mountain of grief. Many people with CF think a lot about life, about timing, about commitments. When one is down in the dumps about one's health, it can often be very difficult to image a bright future.

Another obstacle some people with CF face is the time and energy it takes to be in a relationship. For many people whose health is failing, life can be busy enough trying to maintain their health. This leaves little time to think about what they want out of it. When one is suffering and treatments are constant, thinking about big picture things, like settling down with a partner, often seems out of reach. Not only do people with CF have to deal with the regular complexities of a romantic relationship, but they have to add on top of that the complications of CF.

For myself, these were the thoughts that kept swirling around in my head during the on-and-off relationship that Kim and I had before we finally worked it out. On my best of days, I am an overthinker, but add on top of that the health struggles and disempowerment I was feeling, and I almost threw away the best thing that has ever happened to me.

About a month after the Hawaii trip, I was still trying to come to grips with the disaster that my health had become. Over coffee one day, I made it clear to Kim that our relationship was off and would stay off, so it would be best if she moved on. We had always felt that our problem was a matter of timing and that one day we would be together, but time was now getting on. There was a shared deep-seated love between us, but we hadn't been able to make it work. (Of course, whenever someone says something like this, it usually means that a permanent click is just around the corner.)

However, something changed in the following months of 2007. First, I remember sitting in my living room on a Saturday afternoon, looking out the window. I lived just behind a seawall, and I saw a young couple who had just gotten out of their car and were walking up the hill to the seawall, holding hands. For some reason, seeing this got me thinking about Kim and the idea of a long-term future together.

Big Breath In

Second, about a week or two after this, my cousin and his wife had their first kid. I went to visit them and meet this newest family member. I spent about thirty minutes with them and their new child. During the visit, my cousin asked if I was seeing anyone, particularly Kim. I said that no, I wasn't seeing anyone and I didn't think the whole "Kim thing" was going to work out. But sitting in their living room, holding their newborn daughter and being reminded of Kim, something hit me. *I actually was missing her!* On the way home from my cousin's house, I gave Kim a call, asking if she wanted to grab some dinner at my house and hang out. She agreed. After hanging up and continuing the five-minute drive home, I constructed a plan. I was going to give this one more shot. I would give it a month, and if at the end of that month there was nothing there, I would end it for good. However, if my feelings remained, I would go all-in with the intention of someday getting married. Enough was enough!

It was May 2007, and we were hitting our busy season at the farm, so though time was not easy to be had, I made sure to call Kim as much as I could and we saw each other a couple of times a week. In the evening, she would often come to my place and we would have dinner, go for walks, and she would hang out as I did my physiotherapy. I wanted her to get the full picture of my life as it was. At the end of the month, on Friday May 31, 2007, we were sitting on my front porch watching the sun set over a neighbor's field of budding potato plants, and I shared my plan with her. I told her I had been sizing up the situation over the past month, and after spending this much time with her, I had indeed fallen even deeper for her. I wanted to move forward with this relationship for real this time, knowing it would get serious very quickly.

The final realization for me was this: Kim was the first person in my life whom I'd rather be with than not be with. She was the only person in my life whom I felt more comfortable *with* than *without*.

There was a "completing of myself" when she was around that was missing when she wasn't there. (Yes, I know, how very *Jerry Maguire*-ish of me). This was more than being *in love*; I wanted my life to be hers and hers to be mine, no matter what the future held. I never wanted to be without her.

Kim rolled her eyes and laughed when I laid out my plan (the rightful response to my stupidity), and said she'd figured that this was coming. Anyway, she agreed. It was time to piss or get off the pot. I gave her a key to my house so when I was busy, she could come and go as she pleased. She was amazing, often coming over straight after work to make dinner, then clean up as I did physio. We would watch some TV and then she would head home when I had to go to bed. I'm not worthy of her, not then and not now.

In terms of my health, things stabilized over the course of the spring and early summer of 2007. I felt weak and got short of breath quicker, as I only had about 30% lung capacity, but I was getting by. I had a lung infection in July and went on two weeks of home IV antibiotics. This was not much fun as it was very hot and my PICC line was very sweaty and itchy. But I got through it, taking time off from work and trying to relax, and do the best I could to get myself healthy again.

I mentioned that I had a PICC line put in when I did my IV treatments at home. A PICC line is a semi-permanent intravenous line. PICC stands for peripherally inserted central catheter, and it is a long line that is inserted into your upper arm and then fed through the vein in your arm until the tip of the line sits right above your heart. This is so that large amount of antibiotics can be given to the body without the fear of collapsing the vein in the arm, and it can be done pain-free. All people, when admitted to hospital, have an IV line put in, usually in their hand or forearm. Those who are going to be in hospital for a number of weeks and are to receive high doses of medication, or if there is the potential of doing their IV meds at home, will usually get a PICC.

It is quite the ordeal to have one put in, usually taking about forty-five minutes. The insertion procedure includes loads of antiseptic and an X-ray after the insertion to make sure the tip of the line is sitting is in the right spot. PICC lines can last for up to twelve months; however, the dressing needs to be changed weekly and it cannot get wet. The worst part for me was how itchy my skin would get under the dressing that covers the insertion site. When the nurse takes the dressing off and rubs the alcohol stick over the itchy areas where the dressing was, the feeling is almost orgasmic! The only other drawback, other than the itchiness and needing to keep it dry, is that you cannot lift anything more than a milk jug when the line is in. But based on how sick I was, I wasn't carrying much, anyway.

During this period, I was going into clinic about every four to six weeks, as they wanted to keep a close eye on me. Just as I had tested the long-term relationship potential of myself and Kim, my doctors, throughout the year of 2007, were testing my long-term health potential, paying close attention to what my lung function would do.

As the 2007 harvest season came to an end in October, it was clear that my lungs were not rebounding the way everyone had hoped. I had another clinic visit in mid-November. My doctor and I had a long chat during that visit, and she laid out all my numbers over the past several years. There was a graph with a line showing a pretty slow and steady downhill trend, then a total plummet in November 2006 (Hawaii). The steep pitch back up—the thing we had hoped for over the past year—however, was not there. Instead, there was a straight line moving horizontally out from the bottom of the cliff. The year-long experiment to see if my lungs would rebound had failed. My lung function was not coming back, and there was a real fear that if I picked up anything as bad as I had in Hawaii, I might not have the capacity to make it through. Things were not yet critical, and the doctors thought it might be a bit too early to be waitlisted for transplant, but since things had not improved over the past year, it was decided it was now time for that meet-and-greet with the team at BC Transplant. The referral was made, and after waiting for two weeks, I got a call that an appointment was set for February 6, 2008. My transplant journey now had an official start date.

6.
THE TRANSPLANT JOURNEY BEGINS

"Al slipped in the low gear and let in the clutch.
The truck shuddered and strained across the yard.
And the second gear took hold. They crawled up the
little hill, and the red dust rose about them.
'Chr-ist, what a load!' said Al.
'We ain't makin' no time on this trip."

(*The Grapes of Wrath,* John Steinbeck)

I RETRIEVE MY almost-forgotten 2008 day-planner from the trunk in our spare bedroom. I smell the stale pages holding these remnants of my past, wipe the dust off the cover, and open it to the first week of February. I am surprised by what I find. My memory, more specifically, my *emotional* memory, which is often the most lasting kind of memory, makes me believe that by the beginning of 2008, I was barely hanging on. My emotional memory has me thinking that nothing of significance happened in 2008 other than that it was the year of my transplant workup, the year we decided to go on the transplant wait list, and the year that I had to stop working.

However, as I flip through the forgotten days, I am reminded that less than a month before my first transplant clinic visit, Kim (my fiancée at the time) and I danced the night away at Lynette and Bryan's wedding (my sister and brother-in-law). The Saturday before my first appointment with BC Transplant, I went with my groomsmen to get fitted for our tuxedos for Kim's and my wedding. The night before our first sit down with the transplant doctor, I took a guy I was mentoring out for dessert. That same morning, someone came over to quote us a price for putting in new kitchen cabinets, and the day after our appointment Kim and I had our first pre-martial counseling session!

As I see these appointments chicken-scratched with red ink in my day planner of that pivotal year, the historical memories and thoughts come racing back: What were we doing talking to BC Transplant? Was a transplant really in my future? Kim knew I was sick—she had seen it all first hand in Hawaii—but neither of us really believed that within our first year of marriage I would actually be placed on the transplant wait list.

As I leaf through the pages of the first five months of 2008, there are appointments for doctors and home IV treatments, but those appointments are also buried among other appointments for board meetings, work appointments, social gatherings, wedding parties, and, of course, our wedding on April 26. But let's back up a bit to Wednesday, February 6, at 1:30 p.m. My first meeting with the lung transplant specialists.

This first meeting, as I have mentioned a couple of times, was simply a meet-and-greet. It was a chance for me to get my name on the radar of the transplant program doctors, for them to meet me and Kim face-to-face, and, of course, to physically assess my candidacy for transplant should I need it.

Three primary topics were covered at this first appointment. We first established that my health was failing. It had now been over a year since Hawaii, and my lungs were not rebounding, they were continuing to decline. If I continued on this trajectory, then, yes, there would come a day when I would need a double-lung transplant.

Second, though I was on a downward trajectory, and though my breathing tests had declined below the threshold of when it was appropriate to consider transplantation, based on my quality of life and the strength I still had, we decided that it was still too early to seriously consider expediting the transplant process.

And third, which stuck with me the most, my doctor outlined that receiving a double-lung transplant, at least back in 2008, was not for the faint of heart. What he said was, "Receiving a double-lung transplant is among one of the most difficult medical procedures a person can go through. Waiting for and receiving it will most likely be the most stressful experience of your life. The lungs are the only organ in the body where there is either no living-donor option, or no life-sustaining option to keep you going while you wait. Your lungs need to be working up to the moment of transplant."

Just as important as the physical tests I would undergo to ensure I was a good candidate were the sociological and psychological evaluations. These would ensure I was emotionally, mentally, and socially healthy enough to sustain the live-saving wait for lungs to become available, never knowing if they'd be available in ten seconds, ten months, or never. I'd also need a crucial social support network of family and friends to help carry the emotional load, physically support me, drive me to appointments, and care for me full-time during the immediate months post-transplant.

With this opening volley of information, we decided that with our wedding just around the corner at the end of April, and with my fragile but stable health, we could schedule a follow-up meeting for June and see where things stood then. As we were leaving his office, he said one last thing, "Come prepared to the June meeting with all the questions you might have about transplant. A good part of that meeting will be devoted to getting everything out in the open—both the good and the bad."

Kim and I walked out of the BC Transplant offices knowing that I would most likely need a transplant to save my life. But we also felt confident that day would not be for a long time. We'd get married and have lots of time learning how to live together as husband and wife before dealing with this transplant stuff. So, as best we could, we put it out of our minds and focused on the immediate months to come.

Wedding Bells

2008 was the year of weddings in our family. My sister, Lynette, got married to her husband, Bryan, in January. Our wedding was in April. And Kim's younger brother, Tim, got married to his wife, Heidi, in June. After our February visit with the transplant doctors, Kim and I threw ourselves into our own little world, trying to get me as healthy as possible and, of course, planning for the wedding.

I kept on mentoring a couple of guys at my church. I had CF appointments and follow-up appointments. In March, the fieldwork on the farm once again picked up—I was in my element. Our kitchen cabinets came, I got some dental work done, and somehow it snowed on March 28, but then it turned warm and beautiful with the fresh spring smells in the first week of April. We made the final arrangements for our wedding reception. My dad and I bought a new tractor and some equipment. We went to

The Transplant Journey Begins

an agriculture banquet and, of course, had my stag and drank too much. And then the big day: April 26, 2008.

What do I remember of our wedding day? Well, it is a day that is pictured in my memory through the lens of CF. Our ceremony was a 4:00 p.m. I stayed home by myself all morning to rest. About an hour before pictures, I did some very vigorous respiratory physio, as I knew this was going to have to last me all afternoon, evening, and night. I packed my Ventolin puffer into the breast pocket of my tuxedo and was then off to do pictures before the ceremony. We kept the ceremony quite short and then drove straight to the reception. After greeting everyone in the receiving line, I retreated to the bathroom to take a couple of hits of Ventolin and then finally slumped down into my chair to rest. It was a great party—good food, an open bar, fun games, excellent speeches that had people in stitches and me coughing up a lung, and a pretty good dance.

But after we left the reception, the reality of CF hit once again. I needed to make a stopover at my, I mean, *our* house, to do some physiotherapy before heading to the hotel. I did about forty minutes of physio, trying to clear the hours of accumulated mucus in my lungs. Kim changed out of her wedding dress and into more comfortable clothes, made sure we had everything we needed for the honeymoon, and then we were off to our hotel suite.

There is one memory, however, that the clouds of CF didn't, and could never, touch—and that was Kim herself. The first moment I saw her that day, at the park where we did our pictures, was magic. She was standing on a dock overtop an inlet of water, where the photographers had positioned her for our first meeting. It was a beautiful park where we did our pictures, but the beauty of the scenery was nothing compared to Kim. I walked down a small hill and out onto the long dock. I crossed the fifty-foot distance between us, trying to slow my pace so the photographers could get good pictures, but I wanted nothing more than to run as fast as I could and take her in my arms. She was breathtaking. We spent a lot of time smiling and giggling with excitement when we were able to steal a couple moments alone. Later, as her dad walked her down the aisle, I was so proud of her and that all eyes were on her. Kim hates the spotlight. She has always refused to get on stage with me when I am speaking somewhere, but we did it together that day.

The pastor's message to us was to seek a peace that transcends understanding. We knew that the next years could be difficult. Transplant talk was already underway. So instead of a message about love or commitment, he spoke of peace, something we knew we would need. The only thing that put CF in the background that day was Kim, gazing into her eyes and committing my life to her. Still to this day, Kim is the one person, the one light, which makes all the darkness fade away.

Life after our honeymoon returned to "normal" pretty quickly, with work, physiotherapy, setting up our home, getting rid of material redundancies in combining our stuff, and, of course, more respiratory physio. The months rolled by. As we approached Tim and Heidi's wedding in mid-June, I began feeling worse again, it seemed my lung infections were kicking into gear. On June 18, I had a PICC line inserted; the following day, I began home IV antibiotics, and on Saturday, June 21, Kim and I packed all my medical supplies and drugs, a cardboard IV pole, oxygen tanks, and a small cooler full of IV bags filled with antibiotics, and we headed out for the resort wedding of Kim's brother, about 150 kilometers away. I spent more time than I wanted to during the wedding sitting in our hotel room with antibiotics dripping into my veins while sucking back oxygen to try and lower my heart rate. Because of my medication schedule and just how rotten I was feeling, I had to sneak away to do IVs between the ceremony and reception, and duck out of the reception early. This was life in 2008.

Getting Down to Business

Four days later, on June 25, we had our second meeting with the transplant doctor. Though we were still a little blind to the writing on the wall, he was not. This second meeting had four agenda items to it:
1. The risks of transplant.
2. The life-saving ability of transplant.
3. Our questions about transplant.
4. Next steps on the transplant journey.

My transplant doctor opened the meeting. "What I'm going to do first is talk about all that can go wrong with a lung transplant, basically the negative side of things. You need to know this; take notes if you want. But after today, unless you bring it up, we're not going to talk about this stuff anymore. After today, we're only going to focus on the positives, on the new life that your transplant will one day bring you."

As he said this, I could feel excitement growing in me. For some reason, in talking about the negatives of transplant, it made the process so much more real. I had dreamed about the positives and new life of transplant, but that was all a dream. Talking about the negatives brought a certain realness, a gravity to the situation. Kim was also dialed in. Perched on her lap was the spiral notebook we had brought. Having worked as an executive assistant, she was ready for the onslaught of information about to come our way. With our speechless nods communicating we were ready, the doctor started.

"First, organ transplant is not a cure. What we're doing with transplantation is trading one set of health-challenges for another. The current illness you have is killing you. There will come a time in the not-so-distant future when your lungs will fail; therefore, we have to do something about that. A transplant is your best option. However, a transplant comes with its own set of concerns and difficulties. For the most part, we can handle these things and life will be much better, but still, there is a lot you will need to do.

"Second, you'll still have CF; therefore, you will continue to be followed by your CF team. Your new lungs will not have CF, but you will still need to manage CF in the rest of your body."

Both of these facts were things we already knew. People sometimes take issue with saying that a transplant is trading one illness for another, but this simply means that once someone has had a transplant, it doesn't mean they can take their foot off the gas of being vigilant about their health.

So far, no big surprises. He continued on. "Third, from the moment the new lungs are placed in your body, the clock starts ticking on them. There will come a day when the lungs won't want to work anymore, meaning there will come a day when your body will reject the new lungs. Receiving a transplant is an incredibly unnatural thing. Lung tissue is easily damaged. Therefore, though you'll be taking immune-suppression drugs every twelve hours for the rest of your life, your body's natural defense system will one day begin breaking down these new lungs."

My restlessness began to come alive now. I sat forward so that all my focus was on what the doctor was saying. The fact that my new lungs, if I ever received them, would have an expiration date was news to me, and a tough thing to hear. Our hope, at this point, was that with the proper care and a little bit of luck, I might go sailing into old age. I looked over at Kim, who was hunched over her notebook. She looked up, and I could see the questions turning

The Transplant Journey Begins

over in her mind as well. In my own head, all I could picture was the surgeon placing the donor lungs into my open chest cavity and then hitting the start button on a stopwatch. Kim and I both remained quiet, but I couldn't help but wonder how long the stopwatch would continue to count once I received my transplant.

"Fourth," he said, "though our surgeons are some of the best in the world, there's always a chance, as with any surgery, that you don't make it through surgery. Fifth, the first hours and days after transplant are incredibly delicate, and there's always a chance that your body rejects the lungs outright. If this is the case, there might be very little we can do."

This was something Kim and I had talked about in the lead up to this meeting: the fear of those first couple days. She again looked up from her notebook and glanced at me. We locked eyes, gave a faint smile, and retook our previous positions.

"You will not be able to go back to farming once you have had your transplant," he said. "The environment will be too harmful for your lungs and compromised immune system."

This was also something we already knew but needed to hear from him directly. It was tough to hear, but it wasn't until it became a reality after my transplant that the grief and depression around leaving my first vocational love set in.

"Next, the side effects of the immune-suppression drugs can be severe. We start you on a very high dose of prednisone, an anti-inflammatory, and you may very well be shaking out of your hospital bed in the days after surgery. You'll be three times more likely to develop skin cancer. You'll most likely develop diabetes. You'll need to take blood pressure drugs, and on top of all that, every person is different and there's no way to fully predict how you'll handle the drugs that'll keep you alive. So be prepared."

He paused for a moment, as if searching for something in the recess of his brain.

"Well, I think that's about it . . . oh, one more. If, while you're waiting for your transplant, you're admitted to the ICU or you need to be intubated on a respirator, you'll be removed from the transplant wait list and reassessed once you recover."

The silence that now filled the room was like the silence that leaves one's ears ringing after an arena concert. The barrage of cautionary, mostly fatal information just lobbed our way would take a while to set in. Over the coming weeks, Kim and I would read and reread her scribbled notes. However, we still had three agenda items to go.

After giving us a couple moments to take in everything he'd said, allowing our brains to catch up with our ears, the doctor shifted in his chair. "Now, as I said, that's all the negatives that you need to be aware of. You're more than welcome to talk about them with me or the other doctors at any time, but as I said, I will not be bringing these things up again myself. From here on out, it's only going to be about the positives, because despite all these risks, receiving a transplant is one of the most amazing things that could ever happen to someone in your situation."

I liked this approach. The confidence in which he was showing in moving forward this way, about walking in the hope rather than the risk, planted a seed of confidence in me. After sitting hunched over for the previous couple minutes, feeling the burden of risk that a transplant was going to bring, I shifted positions, sitting up straighter, holding my head up again to meet the doctor's eyes. He paused, looking at us. Kim had a fresh page ready to go for the next set of notes. We looked at each other again.

"You good," I asked Kim.

"Yup," she replied. The doc started again.

"Okay, so, now the good news. Depending on your workup, there's a good chance that the side effects of your meds will be very manageable. You also have no other underlying health conditions other than CF, and that's good. If all goes well, you'll once again be able to travel after your transplant and enjoy an active life like anyone else. You'll be able to work if you want, go for hikes, and basically experience life like you haven't been able to in years!"

As he continued on, I was struck by how calm, poised, and confident he was. There was no hint of arrogance or pride, but a simple assurance based on his many years of experience. He had no notes with him, besides a small medical file with my name on it. The file sat closed on top of the desk he sat beside.

"The chances of not making it through surgery are very minimal. If you can stay as healthy as possible, there's no reason that you won't get your transplant. Acute rejection statistics are very low, and we can often do something to slow it, if you get it."

A warm smile now crossed his face. "You'll most likely have incredible years of health, and there are no limits on what you can do after your transplant." He then finished, "A transplant will most likely be the most stressful experience you'll go through in your life, but it'll also be one of the most remarkable as well."

With the first two agenda items of our meeting now finished—the bad and the good—it was now our turn to ask questions. Since our first meeting back in February, Kim and I had kept a running list of questions. True to his word, he patiently took the time to answer all our questions, even if he had somewhat already covered them. Kim flipped the spiral notebook she had been taking notes in to the front page, passed to it me, and off we went.

How soon after my workup was done would I be wait-listed? Depends on my health. It could be the same day, it could be six months, a year, two years or three years later. Of course, if it was over a year some parts of the workup would need to be redone. Basically, just because we do a workup doesn't mean I need to be wait-listed.

Can someone get more than one transplant? Of a different organ, yes. Of the same organ, yes, but (at that time, 2008) I would need to go to Toronto, as the organ donor rate and supply of donated lungs was still very low in BC.

What is all involved in the workup? I would be given a detailed sheet about what all needed to be done, but basically everything in by body would need to be tested. Loads of bloodwork had to be done, my heart size and pressure measured, my chest cavity measured, and I would have to go through detailed lung tests to actually see what we were dealing with. A bone density scan, carotid artery ultrasound, exercise test, and phycological and sociological exams also needed to be completed. Everything needed to be looked at and tested to make sure I was a suitable candidate to receive such a precious gift.

What if my health crashes before the workup is done? Is there something you can do? No. I could not be wait-listed for a transplant unless I had the full workup done. If I was crashing and had little time left, a full workup would most likely not be possible, thus making a transplant impossible.

Will the post-transplant drugs affect family planning? It was advised to get some sperm into a bank before the transplant, as afterward, how the anti-rejection drugs would affect reproduction would be a bit of a wildcard.

Is there a greater benefit in doing the transplant a bit too early rather than a bit too late? Yes, it is better to do the transplant a bit early than too late. Doing the transplant too late means you are already dead or you are so sick that your body will not be able to survive the surgery. Better to be a bit too soon, giving yourself a better chance at recovery post-transplant. Ideally, however, we want to find the sweet spot of getting everything we can out of your original lungs while making sure there is enough in you to make it through the unpredictable wait and surgery.

How do you decide on whether to do a double- or single-lung transplant? Single-lung transplant was not an option for me. Because the damage to my lungs by CF is infection-based, if they did a single lung, the infection from the remaining lung would just migrate into the new lung, and I'd be no better off than before.

Is there another person with CF who has had a transplant that we could talk to? Yes, they provided support people who had gone through this process before and who would be more than willing to talk to me.

We then came to the final part of our meeting: the path forward. By this point in the meeting, Kim and I both felt we wanted to go ahead and get the workup process started. We gave each other a slight nod and smile as soon as the subject was broached. We had only been married for two-months, but we already knew how to read each other quite well. We agreed that we wanted the workup info on the books, as we knew that my health was declining and we wanted to be prepared. To make a final decision before moving forward to start the workup, my doctor took out his stethoscope and listened to my lungs. He looked at my latest blood work and pulmonary functions tests, had me walk up and down the hallways three times, and then took a reading of my blood oxygen level.

His conclusion was that it might be a bit early to be wait-listed, but he agreed it was better to get the process going earlier rather than it being too late. Over the summer, as an out-patient, I would get the workup done. We then decided to meet again in the fall, once all the test results had been compiled and we had further time to reflect on the information at hand.

Transplant Workup

The workup began exactly two weeks after our visit with the transplant doctor. On Tuesday, July 8, I drove to Vancouver General Hospital (VGH) for a series of pulmonary function tests in order to get a full picture of the state of my lungs. We did about an hour of testing. This turned out to be very difficult given the shape of my health.

Jumping forward to today, now that I am post-transplant, every year, I go for many of these same tests—tests where you breathe in and out (normal breathing), and then on your third breath, you take a *BIG BREATH IN* and then blow all the oxygen out of your lungs as fast as you can for as long as you can, until it feels like your lungs are emptied of every ounce of oxygen in them. Then you take another big breath in, which is often accompanied by a blinding head rush. You then remove the mouthpiece and try to recover as fast as possible before you do it two more times. Other tests include normal breathing through a tube, which is suddenly sealed shut. With nothing to breathe in and no way to breathe out, you need to pant against the sealed chamber for about five seconds. This test measures—well, I can't remember what it measures, but it must do something—and then they open the valve again. These tests go on and on. Being post-transplant, I do these tests once a year as an annual checkup in order to get a broad year-by-year picture of my health, but they are easy to do now and don't take much more than thirty minutes to complete. Back in 2008, with a lung function of around 27%, the tests took well over an hour with a lot of coughing, sweating, and inner pleading for the insanity to stop.

After completing these punishing tests, being constantly out of breath and the blinding headache only increasing with each *BIG BREATH IN*, I had two hours to rest and recover, of which I needed every minute. The next test I reported to that same day was a progressive exercise test. In this test, I had to pedal on an exercise bike with a mouthpiece in my mouth that attached to a tube, which was then attached to a recording machine. The goal was to last for as long as I could on the exercise bike as they progressively increased the difficulty of pedaling. The goal was to last for thirty minutes. This test is so difficult for people in my situation that we couldn't begin until one of the transplant doctors came down to the lab to supervise it.

For the first five minutes of the test, I was feeling pretty good. The lab technician then began increasing the tension on the bike, and I felt the burn, but my heart rate still was under control and my blood oxygen saturation, though dropping a couple percentage points, was still holding. We hit the ten-minute mark, and once again, the tension increased. I held on for a bit, feeling my body heat up, sweat forming on my brow and under my eyes. We hit eleven minutes, and I could suddenly feel it: my heart rate started spiking. At the same time, my blood oxygen levels dropped—93%...92%...90%...88%. All the while I felt myself begin to get smaller and smaller on the bike. My shoulders began slouching, head instinctively dropping, my eyes focusing on my burning legs. As my heart rate went up, my oxygen levels went down. Within a couple of seconds, I felt my legs fading. The transplant doctor who was supervising called it. She removed my mouthpiece and told me to rest and catch my breath while she took a set of vitals to ensure nothing too dangerous was happening inside of me.

When I finally caught my breath and the doctor had a chance to review the data, I asked with a wink how I did. Her response cut to the core of my being, and yet it was also the words I most needed to hear at that moment: "Not very good." Now, don't get me wrong, she is a very kind woman and she was one of my favorite doctors, but she had to tell me the truth in order for the reality I was living to truly sink in. This was not the time to dance around the issue, to tell me lies about my lungs, to give me a false hope that things weren't that bad. The test result, which pointed to me lasting less than half the time I probably should have, was not good enough for her to sugarcoat. I am thankful she didn't. It hurt to hear what she said, but I also needed to begin the difficult work of accepting this was the state of my life. I would not live for many more years without receiving a double-lung transplant. My lungs were just not good enough anymore.

The transplant workup continued three days later. I went to the local hospital and had a full scan of my lungs. This procedure gave the doctor who decides on who gets which lungs one of the two most valuable pieces of information he needed: the size of my lungs and chest cavity.

When it comes to receiving lungs, there are two things that matter the most: blood type and lung size. Gender, race, and age have no bearing on recipient choice. Even the viral infections that one has been exposed to can be overcome with medications, but blood type and lung size are the two non-negotiables. Now, there are stories in very dire circumstances where lungs can be shaved down, or a lobe taken off, but this only happens if someone is on their death bed and a set of lungs become available that no one else can use.

Two weeks after my lung scan, I saw my dentist to get a full checkup so any dental work I needed could get done before the workup was completed. Once I was on the wait list, I could not get dental work unless it was an emergency. Luckily for me, my teeth (and my eyes) have always been the parts of my body that work well; therefore, other than a clean, no extra work was needed.

That same day, July 24, I had a carotid Doppler scan. This is an ultrasound of the carotid artery in the neck. I never really knew why this needed to happen; however, when I woke up from my

The Transplant Journey Begins

transplant and I had massive IV lines coming out of my neck, I understood.

The following Sunday, I was booked in for a CT scan. Apparently, CT scans are in such high demand that the only short notice available time was 8:00 a.m. on a Sunday, definitely the most unique time I have ever had a medical appointment.

Two days later, I was back at the hospital for an abdominal ultrasound, and then three weeks after that back at VGH for a bone density scan, an ECG, and an echo-cardiogram, where they take a close look at how my heart is functioning—mainly its overall size and the size of each chamber. Turns out one side of my heart is slightly bigger than the other, but that is a pretty regular symptom of respiratory disease, nothing unexpected there.

I then had a six-week break from tests. My overall health was somewhat stable at this time, at least as stable as could be for someone who was as sick as I was. The remaining tests were all a bit more invasive, both physically but also mentally.

On Tuesday, September 30, I had my last physical test. It was a cardiac catheter. For this test, I was once again required to lay completely naked and still for a number of hours as a catheter, with some sort of pressure-measuring device on the end, was inserted into a vein in my groin and threaded up to my heart, measuring its pressures.

By this point, I felt I had been scanned and measured neck-to-toe. The transplant team now knew the state of the arteries in my neck, the size of my heart and each chamber, the pressures in and around my heart, and the size of my lungs and CT slices of each portion of them, plus exactly how they were functioning and how far they could be pushed. They knew the state of my abdomen by ultrasound, and they knew how healthy and dense my bones were. The final tests they did measured the only remaining part of my body not yet touched: my mental and emotional health. It was also time for Kim to get into the action, as she had to be part of both these remaining tests. We first met separately with a psychologist and then together with a sociologist.

The sociologist was a wonderful woman. She was soft-spoken, asked insightful questions, and genuinely saw the predicament we were in, and responded with empathy. She was objective, affirming the things were we doing well as a couple, but also calling attention to some things we could work on and consider. Kim and I both walked away from that meeting with a sense of empowerment and encouragement. We knew, no matter what her report would say, that we had been listened to and respected.

Our appointment with the psychologist was anything but empowering. Plainly, the guy was a dick. He seemed to relish the fact that he held my future in his hands, and he straight-out told both Kim and I, in our separate meetings with him, that he had the power to bring this whole transplant process to an end. He basically tried to make clear that his report was the most important one and the only one that by itself could stop all of this. He seemed to be a disempowered person himself and wanted to take that out on us by making sure we felt the same. He outright dismissed and belittled my spirituality and faith background, counting it as a demerit more than a help. He asked his questions with a smug, compassionless expression and seemed to be one of those people who thinks that to show any emotions means you can't be objective. He made Kim and I walk away from our interviews believing that any shot at transplant was now in peril because of the report he was going to write.

Usually, I don't like to write or talk about people in this sort of negative light. And the only reason I do this here is because, in talking with other transplant recipients, I know I was not the only person to have this experience. The guy seemed to relish the idea of casting fear into already fear-filled and suffering people. He

The Transplant Journey Begins

liked to think that he somehow held our lives in his hands as if he were a surgeon. Yet, in reality, I knew my transplant doctor had me sized up pretty well already, and this one report would be just that, one report of many.

A week after these two appointments, I was scheduled to receive all my vaccinations, just to make sure I was up to date, as after my transplant, I could no longer receive any *live* vaccines ever again. It is no problem to get a flu shot, or any mRNA vaccine, but live vaccines using actual virus are a no-go. A week after this, I met with one of the transplant surgeons, where Kim and I learned all about what would take place during the surgery.

The last part of the workup came in mid-November, just a week before our final meeting to go over all the results. This was a consultation with the anesthesiologist, just to confirm my blood type, size, weight, and anything else he needed to know in order to keep me alive during the potential ten-hour surgery.

The tests were now all done. The workup, stretched out over five months, was now complete. I had been poked, prodded, inserted, questioned, empowered, and belittled. Everything was complete; the reports were written and submitted. The transplant team of doctors had reviewed them, and it was now time to meet again. The date was set for November 26, 2008, at 1:30 p.m.

7.
HAZARD AHEAD

"We usually have a destination in mind, but when we get behind the wheel, we expose ourselves to unexpected hazards, as well as unlooked-for moments of discovery."
(*Why We Drive,* Matthew B. Crawford)

ONE INTERESTING PART of being wait-listed for transplant, at least back in 2008, was that once wait-listed, I could not leave the province. The BC Transplant folks said that they could fly anywhere in the province to pick me up if the call came, but due to our provincially funded public health-care model, they could not fly into another province or country. This meant that any out-of-province traveling we wanted to do needed to happen before being wait-listed.

Since getting married, Kim and I had always wanted to do a road trip through the western United States—Idaho, Utah, Nevada, Arizona, California, and Oregon. Knowing we couldn't do this after being wait-listed, we decided to hit the road near the end of October, a month before our final meeting with the transplant team. We felt comfortable doing this, and in our idealist planning, this road trip would line up perfectly with the rhythms of IV antibiotics that we felt my body would need. We ended up cutting it a bit close, as I felt a chest infection brewing as we made our final preparations for the trip, but in talking with my CF docs, they said that under the circumstances, we could go ahead with it, as long as we were paying close attention to how I was feeling and were willing to cut things short should I begin to rapidly decline.

The timing turned out well enough, as when we got home from the two-week trip, it was indeed time for some more home IV antibiotics.

Now, I'm not going to bore you with the day-by-day details of the trip. Suffice to say that no matter what we did, or where we went, my health was the number one factor in every decision. I had all my medications with me, checked and double-checked, and a medical letter from my doctor explaining that I had CF and was allowed to carry all these medications. We also had four large tanks of oxygen in the trunk of the car. At this point, I sometimes needed oxygen to keep my oxygen levels within a healthy range when an infection started coming on. I was also using it from time to time to help me sleep. We thought we were bringing the oxygen to be safe, but little did we know how important it would turn out to be!

Having always lived at sea level, I had never given the idea of traveling at certain altitudes much thought. On our second day of driving, we arrived in Salt Lake City, Utah. Now, I had been sitting in the car all day and had not yet done my afternoon physio, so when I stepped out of the car and walked ten feet, I was done! I felt like there was not enough oxygen in the whole city to get me going. It became apparent that the elevation we were traveling at and would be at for the next couple of days—Nevada and Arizona—would present a problem.

Kim went ahead and looked at the tourist sites while I shuffled along the street, and then I headed back to the car for a rest and a good long coughing fit. When we got to our hotel, I quickly inhaled my Ventolin and did my physio, thus relieving some of the strain on my lungs. But it was clear I was going to be needing a lot of oxygen in order to get comfortable that night.

At this point, we began doing some research into the elevations of the cities we were going to be staying in. I phoned my sister back in Vancouver to ask her to go on the Internet to do some research. We couldn't find all the information we needed with just our map and tour guide books. (This was still before widespread data and hotel Wi-Fi.) It turned out that Salt Lake City and the Grand Canyon would be the only locations that would require oxygen because of their altitude. I would also need oxygen during our stay in Vegas, but that was more due to all the walking and the cigarette smoke in the hotel lobby and casinos.

We stayed in Vegas for three days, the first day walking the strip and the next two spent mostly at the pool or in our hotel room. When we left Vegas, we made for the Grand Canyon. As we turned off the main interstate and headed north toward the canyon, I began getting a headache and feeling lightheaded. The elevation was outside my oxygen limit, and supplemental oxygen was going to be a twenty-four-hour-a-day thing. Luckily, we were only staying one night at the canyon. It was here that the most memorable moment of our road trip happened.

We arrived at around 2:00 p.m., did some walking around, checked out some plaques, and visited the museum. We grabbed some dinner at a local pub and went back to our hotel. After being in the room for about ten minutes, my oxygen regulator, which sits on the top of the oxygen tank and helps regulate the flow of oxygen, began beeping. I took a closer look at the regulator and I saw the low battery indicator was illuminated. This was not something we had ever encountered before, so, of course, we had no spare batteries. To make things even worse, it was a rare-sized battery, the large C battery. So here we were, in our hotel room in a very, very small town on the rim of the Grand Canyon, with a dying oxygen regulator and a twenty-six-year-old guy unable to breathe without it.

Our first thought was to find a phone book and begin phoning around to all the places in the town to see if they were open and if they carried C batteries. It was now 8:00 p.m., and most places were closed. Seeing our options quickly diminishing and knowing that I was not in a state to stay the night at this elevation without supplementary oxygen, we began making plans to leave the canyon and make a dash for Flagstaff. However, before resorting to this final option, Kim jumped in the car and began driving the main street of town, looking for something that was open and could possibly carry the type of battery we needed. Within a couple of minutes, like a phoenix rising from the canyon itself, she spotted a small rundown gas station. As she parked the car and rushed into the shabby convenience store, she said a quick prayer. Without wanting to waste time by looking around, she went straight to the cashier and asked if they carried the coveted C batteries. They did! Kim bought two packs (just in case), hightailed it back to the hotel, and within minutes, hearts pounding and breaths held, the beeping of the regulator went silent and it once again started pulsing normally.

We rounded out the trip in uneventful fashion, staying two nights in Palm Springs, one night in Redding on our way to Oregon, and two nights on the Oregon Coast, before making it home in the first week of November.

It was now only a couple weeks before our final meeting with the transplant team. It was an agonizing decision that lay in front of us, but the road trip we had just taken served as a sign for how tenuous my health was at this time. We were still living in a state of disillusionment, thinking I was healthy enough to go road-tripping throughout the western United States when I was in the shape I was. For me, the whole trip was experienced out of the driver's or passenger-side window of our rented Nissan Altima. The most memorable moments all had to do with my oxygen tanks and the other limitations my health placed on our plans. With the state of my health where it was, we were living life on the edge, only one C-type battery away from disaster. The truth of how close we actually were to being wait-listed had not yet sunk in for us, but one thing we did know for sure, life from here on out was going to be limited, and everything was going to be directed by my lungs.

8.
DECISION DAY

> "At crucial moments of choice,
> most of the business of choosing is already over."
>
> (*Visions of Vocation,* Steven Garber)

THE DAY STARTED out like any other. Kim went to work, and I sat down to my regular routine of physio, with the added routine of home IV antibiotics. This, however, was no routine day, for this was the day that came to be referred to as *Decision Day*. It was the day we needed to decide if it was time to be wait-listed for transplant or not.

All my workup tests were done. The results had been compiled. The transplant team had met to talk about the results and if I was a suitable candidate for transplant or not. It was now time for our voice.

I was on home IV and responding quite well. At this stage in my health, there was a big difference in how I felt *before* going on antibiotics and how I felt when I was *finishing* them. During my sicker moments, I would be yearning for a transplant and saying, "Yes, this is what I need. Give it to me now!" However, after being on antibiotics for a couple of weeks, I would overlook how rotten

I was a few weeks earlier and begin thinking that it was still too early to be wait-listed. This was the mental space I was in as we went into this fateful day.

Kim arrived home from work around noon, and we started out for Vancouver. We drove down the rural road we lived on and turned left onto the highway frontage road. I was feeling good, excited even as the momentum of the day was very much carrying me forward. We continued down the long frontage road for two minutes, came to a set of lights, and turned right onto the connector highway. We made the turn, merged into the left lane, and began crossing the overpass over the highway that would take us north into Vancouver, to the BC Transplant offices.

And then something happened. It was as if something deep inside of me *clicked*. We were driving down the opposite side of the overpass, veering right into the cloverleaf, and merging onto the main highway, when the impact of what we were doing finally and fully hit me: *This would be the day my life would change forever. This would be the day that my wait for a second chance at life would begin. This would be the day I would actually receive the little black pager that could literally beep at any moment, alerting us to the news that a set of lungs had come available. This would be the day the central concern of my life would shift from the disease that was killing me to the hope of new life that a transplant could bring. This would be the day that confirmed I was dying, and the only way out was through receiving a double-lung transplant!*

At that moment, merging onto the highway, having this full truth finally hit me, I turned to Kim and said, "Do you realize we could be coming home with a pager?" From the look on her face, I could tell that, like me, the reality of what we were doing had not fully hit her either. Kim had seen the worst of what CF had thus far served up for me, being with me both in Hawaii and on our recent road trip where she had scoured the Grand Canyon for a battery for my oxygen regulator. Kim was always good when there was something to do or someway in which she could care for me; however, she is very uncomfortable with the unknown. We could always kick the idea of transplant down the road it seemed, but now, being in the car on the way to this appointment with all my workup reports compiled, we were venturing into an unknown future we had no words for. The fact was that there was a very real possibility that within two hours, we were going to be choosing to accept a completely new and unknown path for our life together. The rest of the car ride into Vancouver was very quiet.

We arrived at the BC Transplant offices a little early and sat in the large waiting area. As we sat there, like every other time, we looked around at the other waiting patients and began sizing up the "competition."

Because the offices of the pre-transplant clinic are used for all organ transplant, different organ transplant programs use the offices on different days of the week. By glancing at the others in the office lobby and noting most were coughing, short of breath, wheezing, or on oxygen, one could tell that today was an exclusively lung-day in the office. Therefore, and I admit I am not proud of using this language, all the other patients sitting in the room that day were in some sort of way my competition for receiving available lungs.

On this particular day, most patients in the room were on oxygen. All the little oxygen tank regulators were clicking away as we waited to see the doctor. Each person breathing in their canned oxygen through tubing and nasal prongs. As I scanned the room, I noticed that each of the other patients waiting were much older than I was, looking in their fifties or sixties. I didn't know if this was a good thing or not. I knew people are not prioritized by age, but it still made me think, *Well, if all these people will survive the wait and surgery, I guess I should as well!* Another thing I noticed was everyone looking at me and then, when they thought I wasn't paying attention, whispering to their partner or caregiver. This would often happen to me while waiting at the BC Transplant offices. The look they'd have was usually one of question and astonishment, "What is such a young guy needing a transplant for? How is it that such a young guy is on oxygen?"

I say competition, but that is the kind of dark humor Kim and I would share to get us through these visits and the uncomfortable reality that I was always the youngest person in these waiting rooms. It is, of course, anything but a competition when you are in the company of fellow respiratory sufferers. It's a funny thing, but even though I tend to keep to myself in these medical settings and not socialize with other patients, sitting there with these people gave me a sense of camaraderie. Most were much older than I, and there were only three or four of us patients and caregivers sitting there at one time, but we all knew on some level what the other was going through and how scary and frustrating it was to find yourself in this situation. We all had the same oxygen equipment either with us or at home; we all had, or would have, the tiny black pager on our hip that must go with us where ever we go; and we had all gone through the same gauntlet of tests to get us to this point in our wheezing lives. Though words were rarely spoken, most of us too weak and tired to put in the effort, there was a comfort level with these fellow respiratory travelers, sitting there, oxygen tanks clicking away, keeping a soft and slow rhythm on life's brink.

After we waited for about fifteen minutes, destiny finally came knocking through the sound of the click of a door knob, the swoosh of a door opening on carpet, and my transplant doctor saying: "George Keulen?"

My transplant doctor is a kind and polite man with a gentle voice, but like all good doctors, he has little time to waste, and that day, he got right down to business. Even before leading us into his

Decision Day

office, the first thing he did was have me do a short walking test, something I did each time we met. I would walk the length of the hallway three times, back and forth, then plop down in his office as he would slide the small plastic clamp onto my pointer finger that within seconds would read out my blood oxygen saturation and heartrate. Based on how I was feeling after the short hallway walk, I knew the results would not be good: 88%.

I don't remember exactly how the meeting got going, but within a couple of minutes, he explained that my workup results looked good, there were no red flags, and that I would be a "good candidate for transplant." I admit it was all rather anticlimactic, but on the other hand, I didn't know what I expected. It was then, however, that the paramount question of my life was asked: "So what now?" The final and most life-dependent question of my life hung in the balance.

Now, you might be asking, "How is this even a question?" Was the writing on the wall not yet clear enough for us? I couldn't work, I was on home IV every couple of months, we had just returned from an almost disastrous road trip, and I couldn't even walk the length of a short hallway without becoming short of breath—how is this not a no-brainer decision?

It may seem clear that since my quality of life was complete shit, the decision would be a slam dunk, but in the moment, it is never that easy. Kim and I were on the fence. It came down to the fact that we did not want me to be wait-listed too early. The transplant truth is that there are no guarantees. I was approaching a state where I roughly had a fifty/fifty chance of living for another two years. But once you are wait-listed, that is it, the call could come at any moment.

Second, though my CF body was very fragile, I still *knew* it. I knew how to navigate it, and I knew how it responded. I was walking a very thin line with my health, but I knew it and was comfortable with it. Kim too had learned the ropes of having a spouse with such delicate health, and it was something she had grown comfortable with. Was now really the time to take such a leap? A transplant is something unknown, and it was a scary prospect. Kim and I knew we were not yet ready for the transplant at that moment. If I was wait-listed and by some miracle, the pager began singing and vibrating that night, or week, or even month, we would have been very scared.

Yet, we also didn't want to be wait-listed too late. The doctor had explained that the hardest part of his job was seeing someone who decides to go on the wait list too late and runs out of time before lungs come. He said that because of the situation we were in right now, where my health was stable, he would feel horrible if we ended up waiting too long to be wait-listed and I lost my chance if I crashed and couldn't wait long enough for a set of lungs to become available.

Both Kim and I trusted our doctor, and being at a bit of a loss ourselves, we directly asked him for his advice, knowing that the decision was still ours to make. His vote was to go ahead now, seize the moment instead of kicking it down the field for another couple of months. Kim and I looked at each other. We raised our eye brows at each other as I asked her, "What do you think?" She shook her head slightly and responded, "I don't know." We continued to look at each other as my doctor observed us, trying to discern either a positive or negative reaction to his advice of moving forward with being wait-listed. We both felt helpless, paralyzed by the gravity of the decision and the unknown reality of saying yes.

Then something happened that I never expected to happen, and yet it was the exact thing I knew I needed. There are three doctors at the CF clinic, but over that previous year, the majority of my care was handled by one particular doctor. She knew my case and history inside and out, and she was the one who had referred me to the transplant team a year earlier.

Over the past week, I had wanted to call her and ask her opinion on the whole matter, but my shy and not-wanting-to-bother-anyone attitude—which, by the way, was one of the contributing factors that got me into this premature mess to begin with—held me back from making that call.

As Kim and I sat and contemplated, stumbling over our words and thoughts, looking over the edge of an unknown cliff and knowing that one day we would have to jump, the transplant doctor suggested that he try calling my CF doctor to get her opinion. I was taken aback by this suggestion, and yet an immense sense of relief came over me. This was the last thing I expected, but the most reassuring thing possible. The doctor stepped out of the office. I turned to Kim and said, "Whatever my CF doctor recommends, as long as there is a hint of concurrence from the transplant doctor, that's what we're going to do." Kim agreed.

We waited in silence for the life sentence to come. After about five minutes, he returned to the room. As if listening to a jury report their verdict, I held my breath as to the fate he would speak. He sat down and said that yes, my CF doctor suggested that it was time to be wait-listed. She agreed that though I might feel well enough right now, I had no reserves left if something bad were to happen. My health was failing, my lungs were dying, and it was time to jump. We were in!

Now one would think there would be a lot of paperwork to do once agreeing to such major life-altering decision—an exchange of one's natural born organ for another person's. But there was only one page to read and two places to sign. One giving my consent to the surgery and the anesthetic, and second consenting to receiving blood products and a transfusion if needed.

The largest amount of paperwork came from the cellular mobility company that supplied the pager! We laughed that it needed more signatures to carry around an old-school pager than to receive lungs from another person. We signed all the papers in front of us. The nurse swiveled in her chair to the cabinet behind her and, out of the middle drawer, pulled a well-worn black pager. She then opened her desk drawer, taking out two new AAA batteries. She put the batteries in the pager, turned it on, and set the time and date. After a two-minute orientation on the two-buttoned black box, we found ourselves walking out of the office and waiting for the elevator to bring us down to our car in the parkade, the small black pager hanging off my belt on my right hip. My name was now officially on the wait list for a double-lung transplant, which could come at any moment between now and the moment I would eventually die.

Of the drive home that afternoon, two moments stand out in my mind. The first was my sister calling. The phone call itself was of little significance, but it was my first *pager-scare*. In just having received the pager, it was center of mind, so when my hip suddenly started vibrating, my first thought was, *It can't be!* Of course, in a moment, I realized it was not my pager but my cellphone that was vibrating.

The other thing that sticks out was a conversation Kim and I had about the stress of waiting. As we drove south on Highway 99, heading home, Kim was reading through the transplant manual they'd given us. It said that the main cause of stress during the waiting period is the thought that the lungs will not come in time. We chuckled at this because, as of that point, our stress was still that the lungs would come too soon. However, little did we know that the stress we felt that the transplant would come too soon would be short-lived. Unbeknownst to us, driving home from the transplant offices that day, the stress of our lives was about to swing 180 degrees, from worrying that the transplant would come too early to being petrified that it might come too late!

9.
THE GRAND MINIMALIZER

"Whatever undermines autonomy will be experienced as a source of stress. Stress is magnified whenever the power to respond effectively to the social or physical environment is lacking..."

(*When the Body Says No,* Gabor Mate, MD)

I HAD IT all planned out since the summer. Up until this point, November 2008, having just received my pager, I needed IV antibiotics about every five months. I had been on them in June, when Kim's brother was married, and everything went as planned. I'd started thinking, *If I can hold off on antibiotics again until around the end of November, I'll then be able to get off them halfway through December, gain some more strength, and be feeling great for Christmas!* This was an exciting proposition as the previous Christmas had been a let-down when I had felt absolutely miserable due to issues with hemoptysis and needing another embolization, and of course, the Christmas before that was right after the

Hawaii incident. But here we were, another year down, and I was planning on doing it right this time. In keeping with our plans, on December 4, a week after the big decision day, my antibiotics finished up, my PICC line was taken out, and I was once again tuned up.

Our thinking was that it would be nice if the transplant call didn't come until after Christmas. This way, we could have a comfortable Christmas and then see what the new year would bring. And who knows, I thought, maybe I would even be able to participate in some spring farm work! However, little did Kim and I know that these first two weeks of December, only two weeks into the transplant wait, would be the last time we would ever make plans with a confident assumption that I would be feeling well at any given time.

After coming off antibiotics in early December, I helped out on the farm for a day or two, but very quickly, something didn't feel right. I became short of breath quicker than usual and felt more tired, even when I rested all day. It was clear that the plan of a comfortable-breathing Christmas seemed in jeopardy. My days of security and feeling confident in the stability of my health were darkening, and it seemed my health's downward cycle was picking up.

At this point I should probably explain something about my personality. I am what my doctors call *a minimalist*. This does not mean that I try to live on as few materialistic items as possible (far from it), but it means that I always try to minimalize my symptoms or blame them on something other than the genetic illness that is part and parcel of who I am. I am sure you have figured this out already.

Growing up, I was always quite healthy, so to go from being totally healthy to being quite *unhealthy* was a paradigm shift I

The Grand Minimalizer

needed to adjust to. I have never considered myself to be in denial of my illness. I have always fully acknowledged that I have CF, known it was there, and even taken pride in it at times. I have always faithfully taken my medication and done my physio. But I have always been reluctant in being honest with myself in terms of the restrictions that CF puts on my life. This characteristic, I believe, is one thing that led to my needing a transplant much earlier than I ever would have thought, growing up.

Subconsciously I took steps to compensate for my restrictions, failing to take the time to recognize and name the damage I was doing to myself by living this way. I know others noticed my CF symptoms much more than I gave them credit for, but many people outside our family also just chalked it up to asthma or allergies because I never publicly acknowledged the seriousness of my health concerns. In fact, the reality of what was happening to my health never fully set in for me until the transplant workup was all done and it became a real and distinct possibility that I was going to be wait-listed for transplant.

One night around this time, Kim and I were teasing each other about our body language and nonverbal communication, when all of a sudden, while clearing the table, Kim struck a pose that looked so awkward it was almost grotesque. I instantly knew she was imitating the way I stood. I knew I stood in a unique way that made it easier to breathe, but I'd never realized just how ridiculous it looked!

Before my transplant, while my health was failing, I usually stood with both hands in the pockets of my jeans, leaning on them while also placing pressure on my thighs through the pockets, thus lifting my shoulders off my chest cavity. My right foot would be at a ninety-degree angle to my left foot, with the heel of my right foot resting on top of my left foot. To make this work, I would be bent forward, and my shoulders would be in a bit of a shrugged-forward, hunched-up position, again taking pressure and weight off my chest cavity and lungs. Standing in this position was the easiest and most comfortable way for me to breathe when I was standing. I figured it looked a bit funny, but no more than someone who might slouch, but never did I think I looked that weird until I saw Kim mimicking it. All this is to say that I had been subconsciously compensating for my ability to breathe, even when resting, to where others could definitely notice that something was wrong with me, even while I was still believing I was living a mostly healthy life.

People with CF have an amazing ability to function on very low amounts of oxygen and energy. I always wonder what would happen if someone took my lungs and placed them in a totally healthy person. Would they even be able to breathe? My guess is that to go from normal-functioning lungs to lungs functioning at 25% would feel as if you were choking to death. It is like the frog being thrown into boiling water and being killed instantly instead of the frog that is slowly boiled alive. This is why one of the most effective advocacy campaigns for CF is the challenge of asking people to breathe through a straw for five minutes—this is what CF is like, but for a lifetime.

But back to the *minimalizing*. I struck funny poses to breathe easier rather than notice the fact that I could no longer stand up straight for any length of time. If I was feeling rundown, I would blame it on not getting enough sleep. If I was coughing more and bringing more mucus up, I would think that I could beat it on my own. I was having a very hard time realizing that CF was taking over my life and putting restrictions on me that I no longer had any control over. I kept thinking that if I could just work hard enough, I could get back to an old level of health—do more physio, more exercise, get more rest . . . more, more, more! But working harder and doing more at this point made me go further and further backward. At this stage of the fight, what was needed was not more work and more effort, but rest, allowing the antibiotics to do their work. It meant realizing that the ability to get better was completely out of my hands and was instead in the hands of the supplementary care I was now receiving. Ultimately, it was up to the chances of receiving the gift of life from someone who was roughly my same size, same blood type, and who died in such a way that their lungs would remain perfectly intact while being declared dead.

During these couple of weeks leading up to Christmas 2008, having been wait-listed at the end of November, Kim and I were reflecting on how bad life had become. Here I was, two weeks off antibiotics, and I was already wondering if I needed to go back on them. I spent a lot of time resting in the lead up to Christmas, with Kim doing all the decorating, shopping, and setting up the fake tree she had bought a year before at a boxing day sale (she is always thinking ahead). For the family Christmas parties, I would do my physio before leaving, and then right away again when we got home. When we went to my parents or Kim's parents, I would plunk myself down in a chair or on the couch and wouldn't move too much for the rest of the evening. Kim took the week between Christmas and New Year's off, and I remember that we watched a lot of movies, and didn't go out much. Neither of us were scared that something drastic would happen; we trusted I could make it through the holidays. But like entering the unknowns of being waitlisted for transplant, we also knew that we had entered an unknown stage of the CF journey—the end stage.

The lesson we finally learned during that first month of being wait-listed was that the time for minimalizing was over. We came to see that any control of my lungs was now out of our hands. It was time to rest and to take care of myself as best I could. To do whatever lowly exercise my body could handle and to do my physiotherapy religiously. And as we would soon learn, it was time to head straight to the hospital at the first sign of trouble.

As both my transplant and CF doctor had said, it might be a bit too early to be transplanted, but my respiratory reserves were almost down to zero. If I got hit with something, it could very well be too late. And as I would soon experience, they could not have been more right!

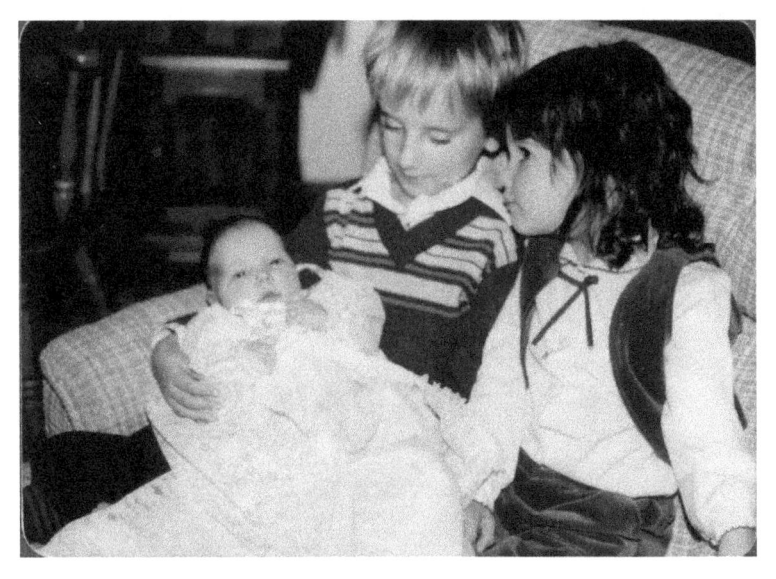

Warren, Lynette, and little baby George

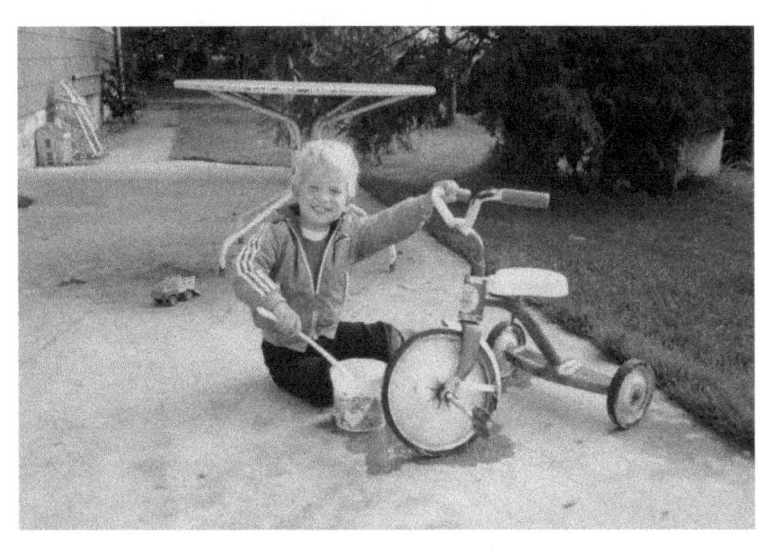

I love my bikes!

Big Breath In

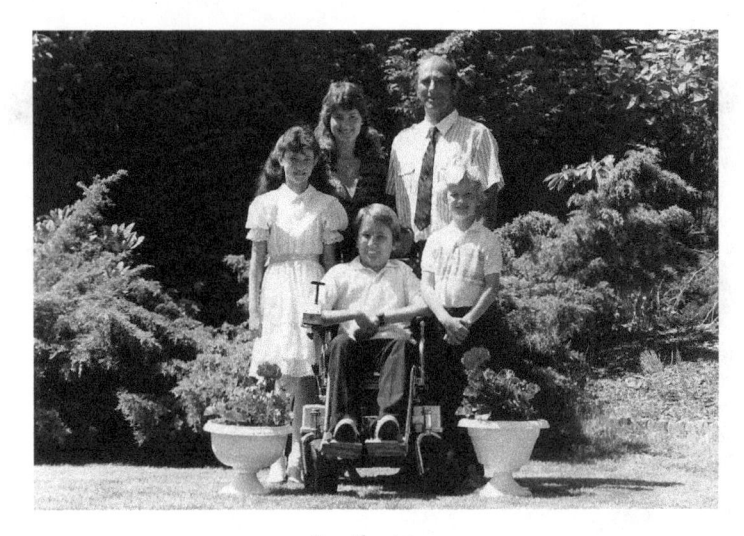

Family picture

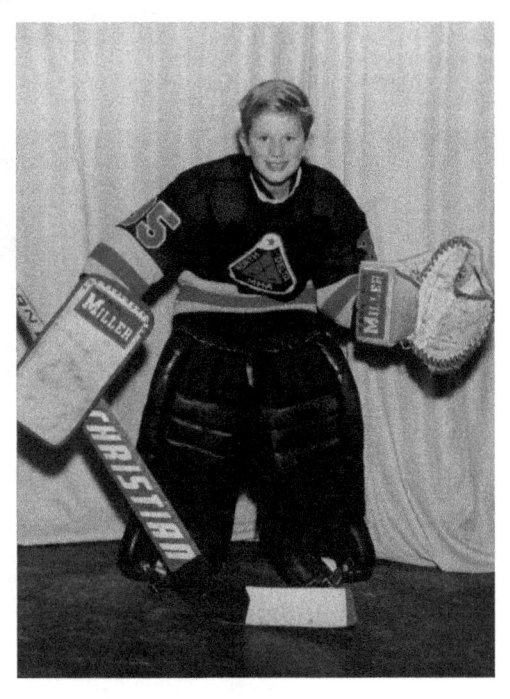

Goaltending, much to my parents' chagrin

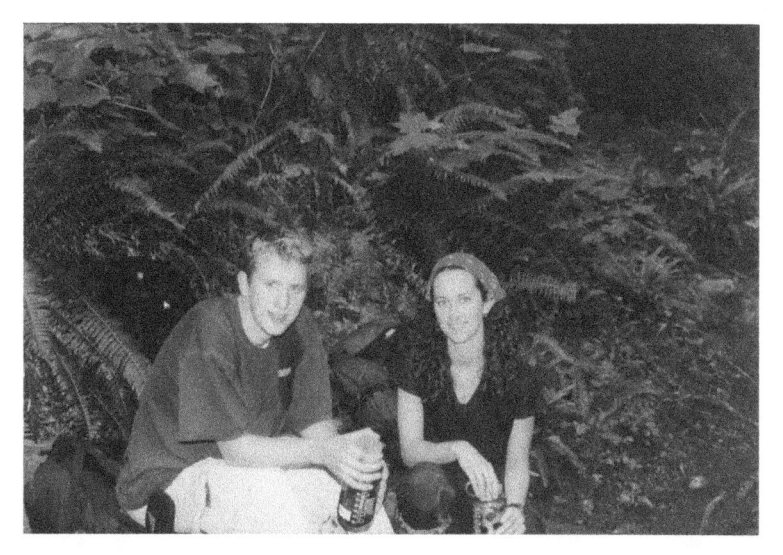

Lynette and I hiking the West Coast Trail

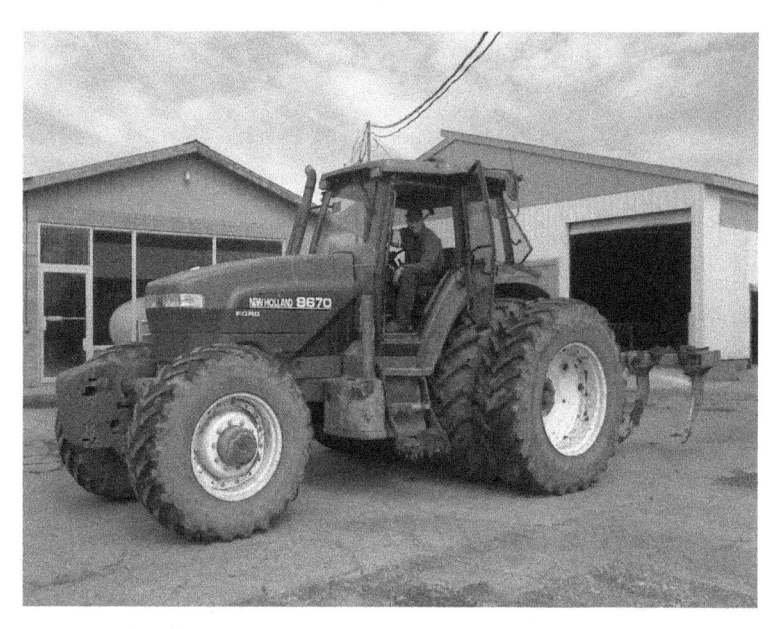

Working on the farm

Big Breath In

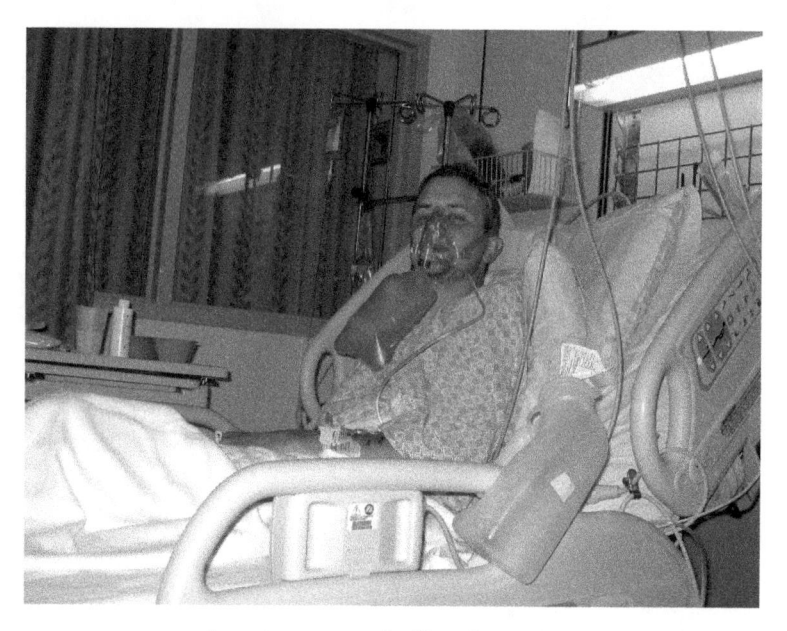

A great way to spend a Hawaiian vacation

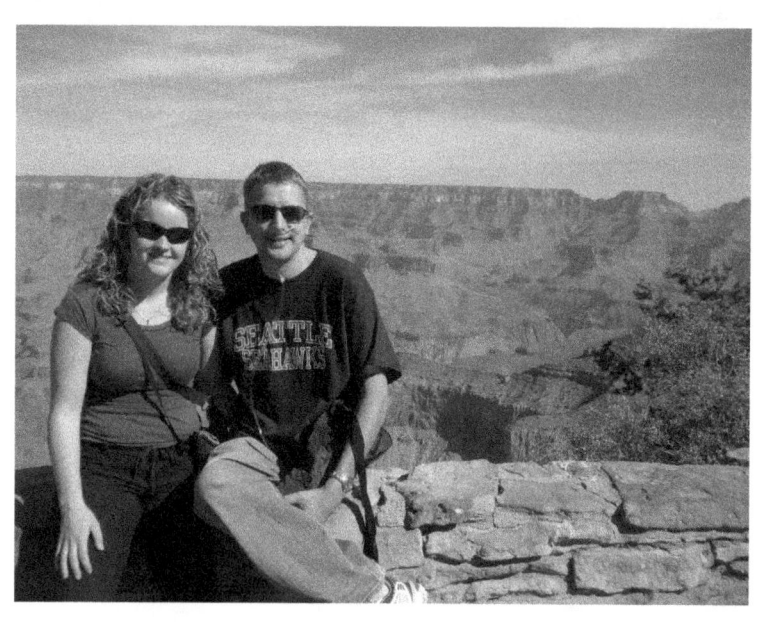

Road trip to the Grand Canyon, with my oxygen tank

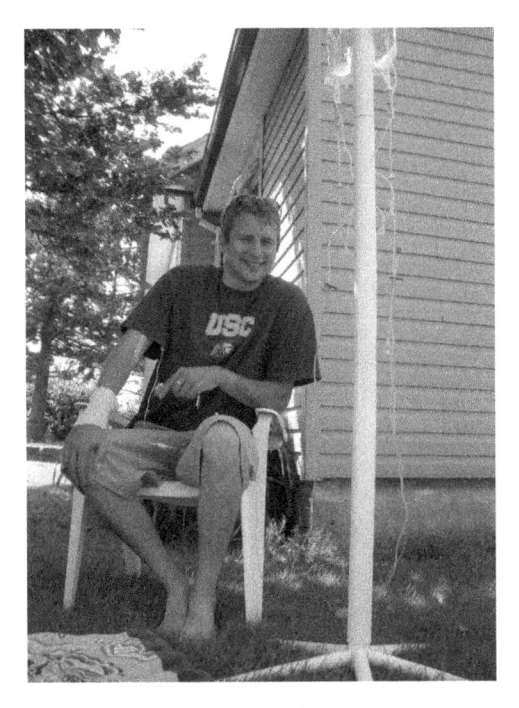

Home IV Antibiotics

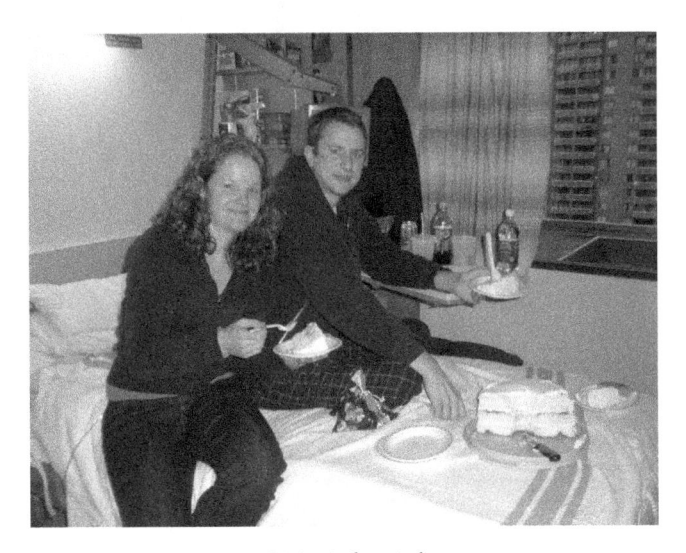

Living in hospital

Big Breath In

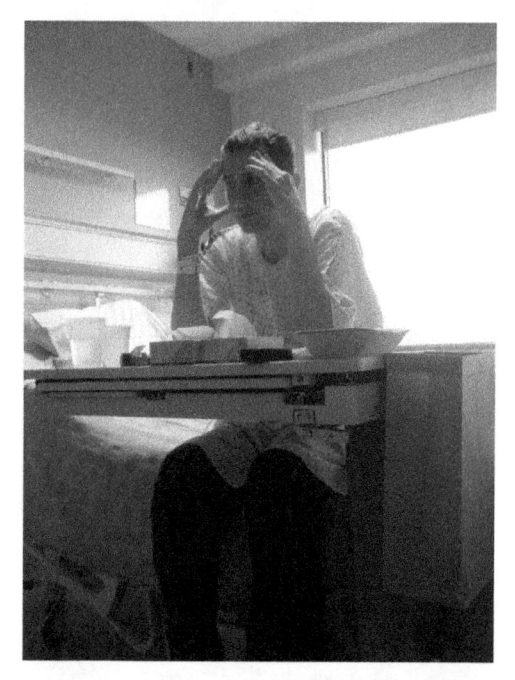

Transplant day: The longest day of our lives!

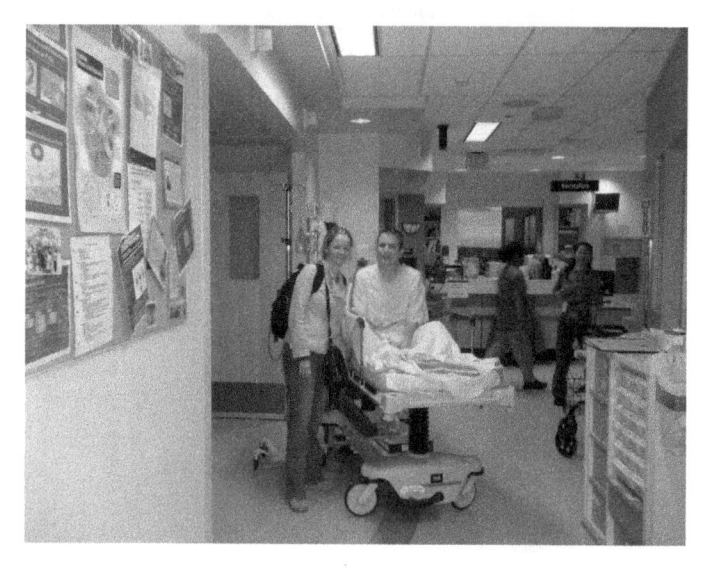

Finally heading down to surgery!

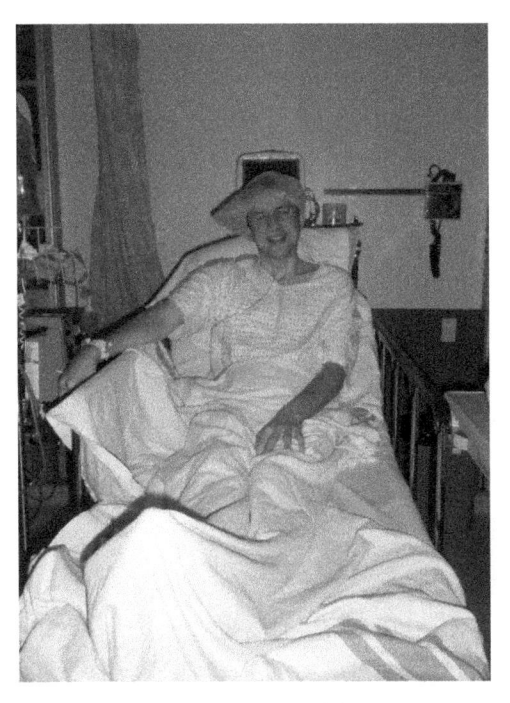

Last picture with my old lungs

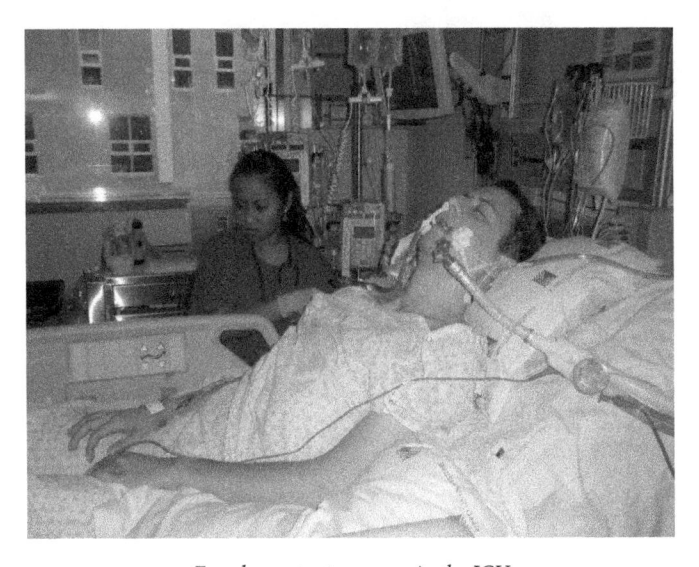

Four hours post-surgery, in the ICU

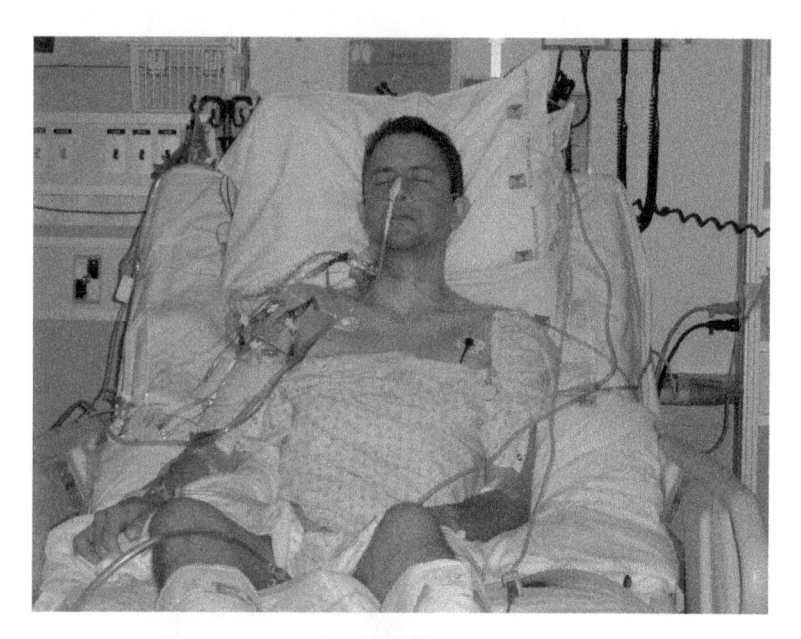

Big Breath In

Resting in the ICU

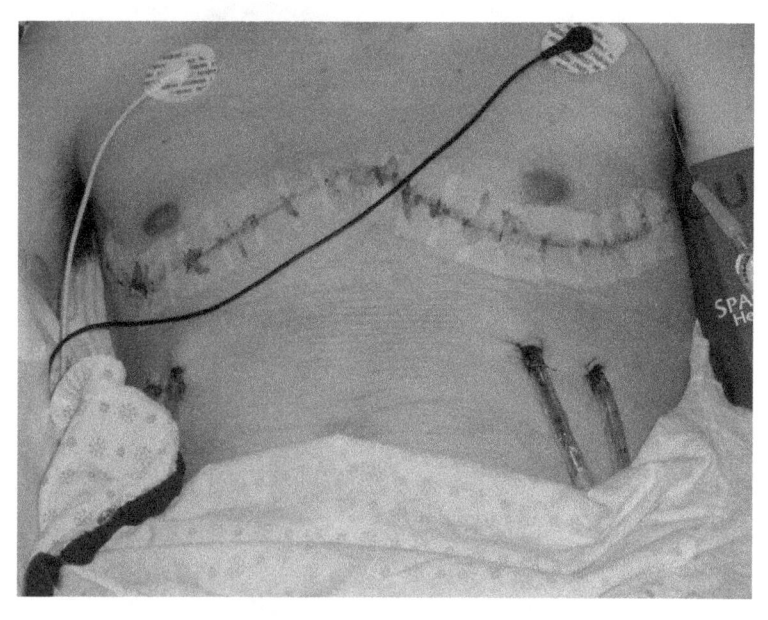

Incision and four chest tubes, post-surgery.

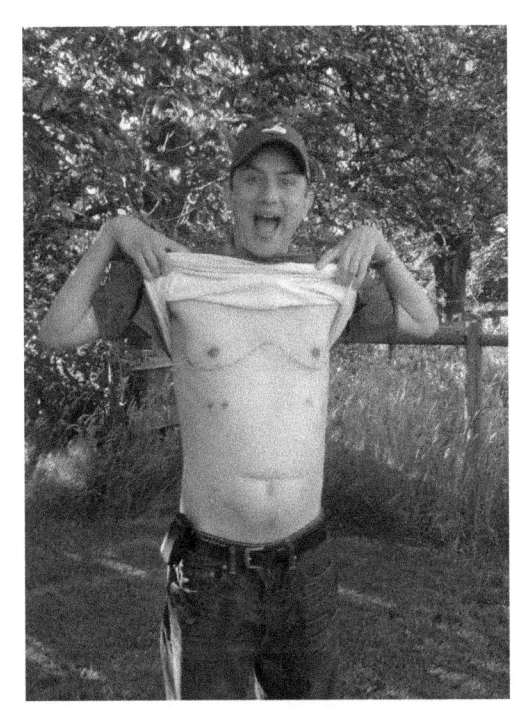

Three weeks post-transplant (incision scar)

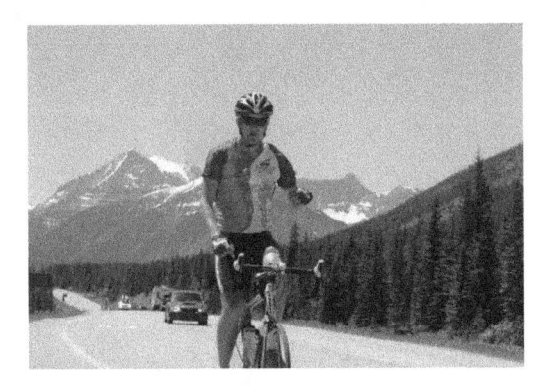

*Cycling across BC
(Gearup4CF fundraiser, 2013)*

Big Breath In

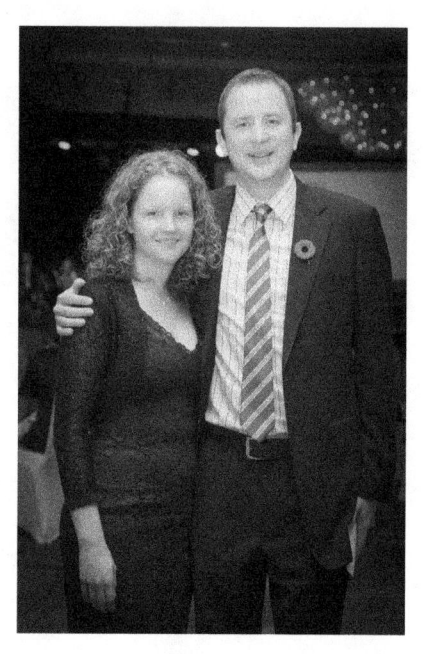

CF Canada Gala Fundraiser, 2015 (picture used with permission)

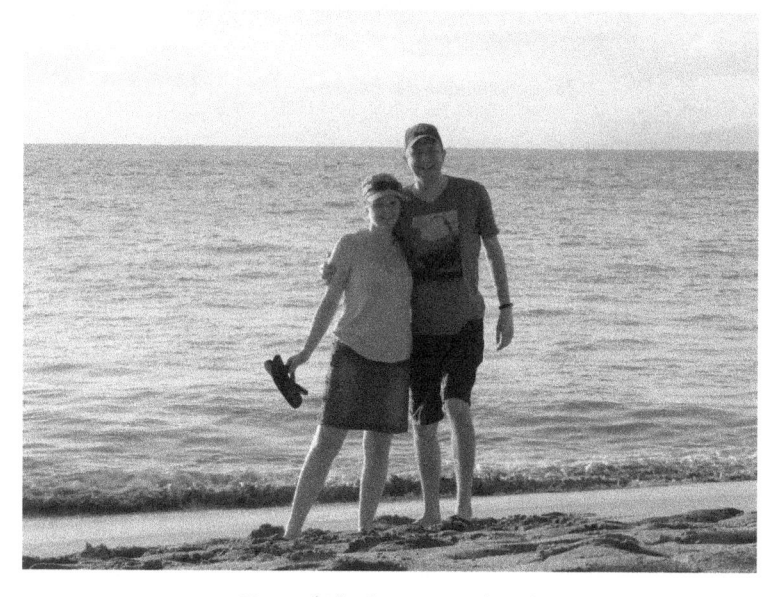

Kim and I back in Hawaii (2017).

10.
CRASH

―

"The second before the sun went out
we saw a wall of dark shadow come speeding at us.
We no sooner saw it than it was upon us,
like thunder."

(*Teaching a Stone to Talk,* Allie Dillard)

THINGS CAME CRASHING down once Christmas was over. I was able to hold off on calling the CF clinic until after the holidays, but with the changing of the calendar year, we knew it was time to get proactive. Of course, what we didn't know was that this was the beginning of the end of my lungs.

With my day-to-day health on an ever-quickening downhill trend, I booked a clinic visit the first week of January. I went to the St. Paul's CF clinic, had an X-ray done, went upstairs to the clinic, and did my pulmonary function tests. After an hour of meeting with the CF team, it was confirmed that I was in the middle of a respiratory exacerbation and I would once again need IV antibiotics.

My doctors set me up on home IV instead of admitting me to hospital. I got my PICC line in and all the antibiotics delivered

Big Breath In

two days later on Friday, January 9. I settled in for two weeks of home treatment and the rhythms of life it would bring. I would go for bloodwork every couple of days at a local lab to monitor my antibiotic levels and kidney and liver function. I would have my PICC line dressing changed every week. However, as I went about these routines, something felt different again. I was feeling more exhausted than any other time I had done this before. The constant schedule of home IV was not allowing me to get the rest I was now needing. On top of this, the antibiotics didn't seem to be kicking in as fast or effectively as they had in the past—I was becoming more resistant.

I got through the two weeks of antibiotics, but the doctors decided it was best to leave the PICC line in case they needed it again soon. They also had less confidence in the effectiveness of this latest course of treatment.

The first weekend went well. I was off antibiotics, rested up, and breathing easier. I entered the following week, thinking things were starting to look up and I just needed a little extra rest this time. But by midweek, something didn't seem right. By Wednesday, I felt myself becoming shorter of breath, and by the time Thursday night rolled around, only seven days after my antibiotics finished, something seemed very wrong. I then began one of the longest weekends of my life, a weekend that consisted of taking in as much Ventolin and home oxygen as I could while also doing my chest physio three to four times a day.

Now, why didn't I call the clinic right away? Well, the easy answer is that I was an idiot! The more introspective answer is that this was not something I had ever done before. I was not yet used to the immediacy of medical care I was now starting to need.

At this point, I figured it was the infection coming back, that I was once again going to need antibiotics. This was certainly not worth showing up in the ER on a weekend, with no CF doctors around, and risking all the other infections I could pick up there. No, I would wait it out at home. After all, first thing Monday morning, I had a scheduled clinic visit where everyone would be expecting me and where I would get all my tests done in proper order. I figured the worst-case scenario was that I would end up in hospital for another round of antibiotics—but nothing more than that.

Monday, February 2, 2009

With the weekend now over, I was actually looking forward to my clinic visit. Things had become *that* uncomfortable. For four days, my lungs had felt like two large rocks sitting in my chest. Although I had accepted the fact that I was going to need a transplant at some point, the delicate state of my lungs and health I had not yet fully comprehended. However, this day will go down in my personal history as the day my health-bubble was officially burst. In the days leading up to this clinic appointment, any sort of excursion—and I mean walking the ten steps from the front door to the car—sent me into a near panic as it seemed my lungs could not get any air in. Whereas before it felt like my airways were skinning straws, it now felt like my lungs were solid masses, not wanting to take anything in or let anything out.

I had joked over the weekend that I must have a collapsed lung or something because of how short of breath I was and the weight I was feeling in my chest. To be safe, we had researched the symptoms of a collapsed lung, but it would always mention an immediate shortness of breath accompanied by a lot of pain. Neither of these boxes checked with my experience, and so I carried on, waiting the four days for my clinic visit.

Big Breath In

In our driveway, as I was heading out to my clinic appointment that morning, I knew I was in real trouble. I had not even walked the fifteen feet to my truck when I was already gasping for air. I had to stop, lean against the hood of my truck, and try to take some deep breaths before I could even get my keys out of my pocket to open the truck door. Another ten minutes later, while driving down the highway, I was slumping forward, holding onto the steering wheel with both hands, trying to lift the weight of my shoulders and rib cage off my chest, trying to suck as much oxygen into my lungs as I could. I had no doubt I would be staying in the hospital that night.

I got to St. Paul's in the regular forty minutes it takes during light rush hour and parked in the underground parking. I hobbled my way over to the elevator, roughly 200 feet from where I parked, assessing how I was feeling compared with all the other times I had made this trip. All I knew this time was that by the time I had walked 50 of the 200 feet, I already had to stop and rest, bent over with my palms on my knees. It felt like I had run a marathon. A couple of minutes later, I finally made the elevators. I got on, punched the main floor button, but instead of shooting straight up, it stopping on the restricted floor. As it did, I almost let out a cry of agony as this short stop would add another twenty seconds to the time I would be able to find a place to sit down.

The elevator stopped, and lo and behold, a nurse from the CF clinic got on. She looked at me with what I could detect was a half-smile of concern and asked in a casual way how I was doing. I said, "Okay, but not the greatest." Much to my relief, she left the pleasantries at that as the elevator once again got going and came to a shuddering halt on the main floor. I shuffled off, telling my CF nurse I would see her upstairs after I got my X-ray done.

The X-ray lab was a good hundred feet down the hallway, a trip I had made many times, but it was now the longest hundred feet

I had ever walked. I made my way into the X-ray reception area, looking as strong and confident as I could, and slumped down in the chair beside the reception desk. Now that I was sitting, I was able to catch my breath a bit easier and was looking at least half normal by the time the receptionist came to get my name. I shifted chairs over to the waiting room and rested for about five minutes before the X-ray technician came to get me.

As soon as I stood, walked down a short hallway, and through the thick double doors where the X-ray machine was, my shortness of breath returned. I knew I was not looking good, and I felt ridiculous as I stood there watching her set up the slide and get the machine ready. I was hunched way over, sucking in air, not even able to stand up properly.

An X-ray can be total torture for people with advanced lung disease. Each time a picture is taken (two pictures are always taken for a chest X-ray, one from the back and another from the side), you need to take a big breath in and then hold it for about five seconds. With the state I was now in, I breathed in what little air I could, but right away, this sent me into a coughing fit. I wasn't breathing in enough oxygen to even last me for five seconds.

Somehow, she got the two shots she needed, but told me to wait for a moment as she checked the quality of the images. I had gone through this process many times before, but now I was squatting in the middle of this large X-ray room. I was mentally willing her to hurry up and come out from behind her protective booth to tell me the shots looked good, thus sending me upstairs to see my CF doctors and hopefully get some answers and treatment for what was happening to me. I could tell she was taking a second and then a third look at the X-rays. She then stepped back out of her booth, and instead of coming back into the room where I was suffering away, she went to a room farther back, seemingly to confer with a colleague, but no one else was around. After a minute, she emerged from behind her booth and asked, "Are you seeing a doctor here in the hospital today?" I told her I was going up to the CF clinic as soon as she was done. She then confirmed, "So you are not leaving the hospital now, but you are going to see your doctor here, in *this* hospital?"

"Yes," I replied. "I am a CF patient going to the CF clinic on the eighth floor." I now knew there was something very wrong with my X-ray.

She said again, "So you are not leaving the hospital, and your doctor, who is in this hospital right now, is going to see your X-rays right away?"

"Yes. That is exactly right."

She nodded, looked at me with contemplating eyes, began to turn back, thus allowing me to leave, but then quickly turned to face me again. "I am not supposed to say anything to you as I am not allowed to discuss the results of your X-ray, but I do feel I have a moral duty to tell you. According to your X-ray, it appears you have a collapsed lung! Please, do not leave the hospital under any circumstances without first talking to your doctor and making sure your doctor sees these X-rays. I will call around and make sure they are reviewed right away and try to get ahold of your doctor upstairs, but my advice is to go straight upstairs to your clinic and hopefully, by the time you get there, they will already know. You must go straight there."

As she said this, I was struck with deep fear, but I also did not respond with the panic one would think. (That would come later.) The technician said all this in such a way so as not to confirm it, so I was able to remain calm and hold onto the faint hope that maybe a mistake was made. However, deep down, it was the only logical explanation for what I was feeling. On the positive side, at least it meant I would receive immediate treatment, bringing relief sooner rather than later.

I started again for the elevators, the technician's gaze following me down the hallway. I now knew the answers to what I was dealing with were floating through the digital records of the hospital system and would soon be seen by the proper professionals who could do something about it. The elevator I staggered into arrived on the eighth floor, and I hobbled my way down to the CF clinic at the end of one of the wings. For some reason, now that I had an idea of what was going on, I felt more determination in my step, not as deflated in terms of how I was feeling. The glimmer of a fighting spirit began taking shape in me.

It turned out that I had beat the news of the collapsed lung upstairs, as the clinic administrator showed me to my exam room and told me to wait. The technician who does the pulmonary function tests, which are usually the first thing you do once you arrive at the clinic, came in and gave me two hits of Ventolin and told me she would be back in five minutes to do my lung tests.

At this point, I began to question how fast news could travel in a hospital. I figured if I did indeed have a lung collapse, I should say something to the PFT technician so that I didn't go and do my blows, thus making the collapse even worse. On the other hand, I was also curious about how bad my lung function was at this point; therefore, I figured I would go along with whatever came first (curiosity often wins out over common sense with me).

I sat hunched over, feeling a bit of reprieve as the Ventolin hit my airways and they began to expand a little. I was able to straighten up slightly, at least enough for the PFT technician not to be tipped off that I was on the verge of disaster. She came back five minutes later, prepped the small machine that would measure my lung function, and was about to hand it to me when, without warning, one of my CF doctors came through the door, took one look at me, and told the PFT technician to stop all testing. Without waiting for the technician to leave or ask how I was doing, she confirmed that

Big Breath In

I had a collapsed lung and needed to get down to the emergency department right away to get a chest tube. Apparently, critical news *can* move pretty fast in a hospital; I had only been upstairs for about eight-minutes.

At this moment, however, time seemed to stand still with the confirmation of my collapsed lung, the look of concern in my doctor's eyes, the realization that it was so serious that the clinic couldn't do anything for me and an emergency response was needed, and those words I had never really heard before—*chest tube!*

The PFT technician packed up her things, wished me all the best, and left the room. My CF doctor explained that a porter was coming with a wheelchair to take me down to the ER and that she would check in on me in the afternoon once the chest tube was in. Before she left the room to make some more calls, she said she would try find a bed for me on the CF ward after the chest tube was in.

All alone in the exam room, the words "chest tube" ringing in my ear, it all became too much. For the first time in his whole journey of declining health and being wait-listed for transplant, something snapped inside of me and I broke down crying. *How did I get myself into this? What does this mean for my transplant chances? Will I ever return to my normal lung function range?* It felt like my reckoning had finally come. It was the final dagger to any illusions of safety and stability I had in my lungs. It was this moment, sitting alone in exam room six, waiting for a porter to pick me up in a wheelchair, that the fear my transplant would come too soon made the violent U-turn to a despair that it might not come in time.

I made a quick call to Kim, who was already at work and not aware of how bad things had gotten that morning. She was now on her way to the hospital. I also called my parents. My dad picked up the phone, and as I began telling him that I had a collapsed lung, I broke down in tears again, sharing that I was going to need a chest tube. He passed the info to my mom, and she too was soon on her way to the hospital.

Within ten minutes, the porter arrived with a wheelchair and wheeled me down the long hallways, down the elevator, and past the X-ray room where I had been hobbling around some thirty minutes earlier. I was wheeled to the far end of the hospital, from my quiet exam room eight floors up to the bustle and noise of the packed ER.

I was brought into a very large room, moved onto a bed, and curtains were drawn around me with other patients only about eight feet away from me on either side, each with their own curtains drawn around them. With my health so fragile and knowing I was only one serious infection away from being in even worse trouble, not to mention the unknowns of the impending chest tube that was going to be stabbed into my chest, this ER was the last place I wanted to be.

I lay on my back, turning from side to side every couple of minutes, trying to catch my breath and slow my breathing and heart rate. It didn't take long for a respirology resident to come see me. He asked me how I was feeling, told me he had already seen my X-rays, and took a quick listen to my chest and the lack of breathing capability in my right lung. He finished with a quick set of vitals and then explained what was actually happening inside of me.

The medical term for what I was suffering from is *pneumothorax*. Due to the state of my lungs, my right lung had developed a small hole in it. Having a small hole in your lung means that air can escape the lung, but it then gets stuck between the outside of the lung and the chest cavity, in what is called the pleura. When air gets into this space, the pressure outside the lung becomes greater than the pressure inside of it, thus collapsing the lung. The X-ray showed that I did not have a total lung collapse on the right side, but over half of it was indeed down. To correct this, they would insert a small tube through my right pectoral muscle, between two of my ribs (please, dear God, don't hit a rib), and into the chest cavity where the air was sitting. This tube would act as an escape route for the trapped air, thus relieving the pressure outside the lung, automatically allowing the lung to expand to its normal size.

The only thing that would prevent this was if the hole in the lung was too big and air continued escaping; however, they would know this right away as the lung reinflation would be almost immediate once the chest tube was in the right spot.

They said they would start with a small tube, hoping this would be enough. They could move up to a much larger one, which would also be more painful, if it was needed. Kim and my mom had both arrived to hear how things would go. Being a former nurse, my mom was relieved to hear that they were first going to try a small chest tube, as she had seen and taken care of people with large tubes and knew how painful they could be when going in and how uncomfortable they would be after. (As an aside, coming out of my transplant surgery, I had four of the large chest tubes, and I still possess the scars from them.)

After everything had been explained, I took some Ativan to try to take the edge off before the procedure. Unfortunately, it didn't work very well. I came to learn at this time that I have a high tolerance for pain and anxiety medication.

It was thirty minutes later that Kim and my mom were asked to wait outside the curtain. The team who was going to insert the chest tube was made up of the medical resident I had already met, a respiratory fellow (supervising doctor), and a medical intern who was observing this procedure for the first time. The fellowship doctor explained the procedure again and had the resident give report on everything he knew about me. He explained that since St. Paul's is a teaching hospital, he was going to be supervising as the resident would perform the actual procedure. Their practice in teaching moments like this was to observe once, do one under supervision, then begin doing it on your own. This medical resident had already observed one; now, it was his turn to take it on himself under supervision.

Having a chest tube put in is not the most difficult procedure, but it also isn't a walk in the park. There are many things that can go wrong, including needing to be intubated, creating a worse collapse, or severe bleeding in the lungs; therefore, the doctor who was supervising was very stern with his instructions. From my point of view, this was both a little comical and scary.

It began with the unwrapping of all the sterile medical supplies they would need to do the procedure. To get the tube in, they had a hard-plastic needle (it looked like a knitting needle) that had a very sharp point on the end of it. Around the outside of the needle was the pliable chest tube. Once the sharp point of the needle pierced the skin, muscle, tissue, and chest wall, it was retracted, leaving the small chest tube in place for the air to escape. First, however, they have to make a small incision so they don't tear the skin when they start applying brute force to puncture the chest.

With all the sterile materials unwrapped, they were ready to begin. The resident took a syringe of freezing and inserted it around the area where they would make the small incision to help get the chest tube in. As he was putting the freezing in, I began wincing and moaning a little bit because of the stinging. It was at this moment that the junior intern, who was observing, looked down with compassion and said, "Don't worry. This freezing is the most painful part."

My spirits lifted. I had been preparing myself for this to hurt like a son-of-a-bitch. But as quickly as my spirits lifted, they fell to

Big Breath In

the floor as the supervising fellow snapped his head in her direction and said, "That is not true. Don't ever lie to your patient." He then turned to me and said, "I am sorry, but this is going to hurt a lot, much more than this freezing."

"Great, thanks!" I winced back to him. I smiled a futile smile, but I also appreciated the frankness of the doctor. I like the straight facts when it comes to my health. I would rather be able to prepare myself for whatever is coming, even if it is going to be painful, than be surprised when the pain hits me.

The freezing was in, it was taking effect, and in a minute, the small incision was made. At least I didn't feel that! The medical resident then took the long plastic needle with the sharp point on the end of it, and though I couldn't see or feel it, he placed the sharp end into the small incision. What happened next would have been quite comical if it didn't hurt so much. With this being his first chest tube insertion, the resident didn't know how much pressure he would need to apply in order to puncture my muscle tissue. I could tell he was beginning to put pressure on the tubing as I could see him leaning over me, and I began to feel pressure on my chest, but nothing was happening. This went on a for a couple of seconds as the pain increased. The supervising fellow began coaching him, reminding him of what he had to break through, but also to continue to be aware of where my ribs were and make sure to not hit one. (*Oh shit!*). As I was looking up, I could see stress and self-consciousness in his eyes. The needle began to bow out in the middle as he was applying a lot of push at the top, but it was not breaking through.

He stopped, and they made a bit of a deeper incision with the scalpel—I felt that one! The resident once again placed the pointed tip of the plastic tubing into the incision and felt for my ribs, which he was aiming to shoot between, then with more pressure than before, came down on the needle. *Poof!* Straight through the chest wall it went, and wow, now I knew what they were talking about. It was one of the most painful things I had felt up to that point, and yet, in that moment, there was also the feeling of relief, as my breathing became a bit easier.

The needle was quickly retracted, leaving the small hollow chest tube behind. The supervising fellow put his ear to the tube—he could hear air escaping through it. It was difficult to get it in, but the resident nailed the spot perfectly. The tube was stitched in place so it wouldn't move, the surrounding area was packed with gauze to absorb any fluid or blood, and within twenty minutes I was packed off to X-ray once again to make sure everything was in the right place and to so see if anything had changed yet in my lungs.

The X-ray looked good. The tube was then hooked up to a suction machine, and I was moved into an individual room up on the CF ward. Over the next 24 hours, I could feel my breathing getting easier as the chest tube worked exactly as it was designed to, removing the air and fluid outside the lung in the chest cavity, thus allowing the lung to expand more and more.

There was some back and forth about how long I would need to be in hospital, but since this was my first pneumothorax and it seemed the hole was quite small, if the suction slowed and no more fluid was coming out, only a couple of nights in the hospital would be needed. Sure enough, within a couple of days, it seemed that I had returned to normal. It actually didn't seem like there was a chest infection at this point; my lungs were just very fragile. The clinical team thought that I might as well be discharged once the tube was pulled. They removed the chest tube on Friday morning, and by that afternoon, only four days after hobbling into the hospital, I was discharged and feeling much better.

There were three significant events that happened during that hospital stay that would shape much of my thinking and experience going forward in my transplant wait. First, I had what one might call a spiritual, mystical, or if you don't want to go down that road, a hopeful premonition. Around 2:00 p.m., on my second to last day of hospitalization, I was standing between my bed and the bathroom door, looking out the window of my room. I was standing at about a 45-degree angle to the bed and window when all of a sudden, a deep confidence hit me, *I will get my transplant!* Being a person of faith, I tried to stay in the moment for a couple of seconds, testing the spirit that seemed to confirm something deep within me. In doing this, an incredible peace and confidence came over me. *I will be getting my transplant.* This feeling struck me to the core of my being like nothing else had, later helping me persevere at the worst moments when I thought all my waiting was hopeless.

A second reality came alive in me during those five days of hospitalization that was based much more on science and empirical data: *I was going to be hospitalized more and more.* My days of home IV were coming to an end. A retired CF physiotherapist named this reality for me. On my second full day in the hospital, when she was filling in for my regular physio, she came to check in on me. We were chatting about the state of my health and then she stopped. She looked me straight in the eyes and told me it was time that I needed to start coming into the hospital when I was sick. What I needed now more than anything when I had a respiratory exacerbation was rest, and the only place I could get the rest I needed was in the hospital. I needed to smarten up, get over whatever it was that was preventing me from submitting to hospitalization, and begin taking seriously the state I was in.

I hold an incredible amount of respect for my CF physiotherapists, and so when she spoke these words, they hit hard. There was no more time to put hospitalization off. I had to wake up to the truth within me, one that everyone had been trying to point out for years, but that I had been too stubborn or scared to see. The hospital would become my second home, a place that I needed to become more comfortable with. I was going to need the rest and care that only an institution of caring and professional people could provide when things got bad.

Third, it was made clear to me during these days in the hospital that lung collapses and lung transplants do not go well together. In fact, they are quite antithetical to each other. Pneumothoraxes can often complicate the lung transplant surgery, and enough of them can almost make a transplant impossible. If enough mucus escaped the lungs and got stuck between the chest wall and the lungs, it could form a strong adhesive, one that could cause real harm to the chest cavity during transplant surgery. In addition, the scar tissue that would form between the lungs and chest cavity, and the increased damage to the lungs, would make lung removal very difficult, thus endangering my life during surgery, but also my own life expectancy before transplant could be decreased with the rapidity of scar tissue formation in and around the lung. Whichever way it might affect me, I was warned that I would need to be very careful about lung collapses, and in the acute phases of infection, I had to try to control my coughing—not to cough less, but to keep it in control, as my lung's elasticity was becoming restricted.

Thus, after this hospitalization, and up until a month after my transplant, I lived with a healthy fear and respect of another collapse. Like a separated shoulder or concussion, once you have one collapse, it only becomes easier and easier to get another.

Being in hospital for those five days seemed like a long time. I had not been in the hospital for any length of time before, other than Hawaii, but of course that was different. Even though Kim was able to visit each day, we were both glad when I came home, as we hated spending our nights apart. However, little did we know that this four-night hospital stint would be the first (and shortest) of many more over the next seventeen months.

On leaving the hospital, I was told I needed to take it very easy. Coughing had to be done *lightly*, and I was not able to lift anything that would cause my lungs to be exerted or my blood pressure to go up for at least a week.

I still had my PICC line in from January, so the following Sunday morning, I had to go to the public health clinic to get the dressing changed, and on Monday, I had to get some blood work done for a medication they had started me on named Tobramycin. This is an especially potent drug, one they usually held in reserve until someone really needs it, as it comes with some pretty nasty side effects. I didn't experience any of the side effects at the time. However, by the time of my transplant, I was having permanent hearing loss in my right ear because of this drug (the benefits of being on the drug outweighed the lifelong side effects; therefore, I welcomed being on it later.)

After the weekend, I had my bloodwork done, and the following day, I had a follow-up appointment at the CF clinic. Throughout most of my childhood and early teen years, I had been a pretty anonymous patient at the CF clinic. But by this point, as I rounded off my twenty-sixth year, I was becoming more and more popular: first, as the guy who went to Hawaii and almost died; second, as the one considering transplant, then as the one now wait-listed; and now third, as the guy who walked around for four days with a collapsed lung. During one of my clinic visits around this time, I found myself standing outside the administrator's office of the clinic, and I was looking at all the files that lined the shelves behind her desk. All the charts had multicolor tabs with a three-letter coding for reference. I saw one right near the middle of the pack, and it was a very large file. I made note that the first letter on the chart was a K and then noted the colors of the tab. About twenty minutes later, as I was sitting in one of the exam rooms, the doctor came in carrying that very large file, the one I'd focused on as being one of the largest on the shelf. Coincidentally, as he came into the room carrying my chart, the whole first section of the file fell out and onto the floor. He apologized and said, "It's about time we thin your file."

I replied to him, "A file that size is usually a bad sign, isn't it?"

He feigned a smile and answered, "Well, it isn't a *good* sign."

But this is the way it goes when one begins to get this sick. More trips to the clinic, more bloodwork, X-rays, CT scans, PFTs, and other reports, all of which tend to create a thick juicy file for the reading, and of course, you become front and center with everyone on the clinical team. If this wasn't enough, though, my reputation and popularity around the clinic were going to jump one more notch.

I had my follow-up clinic visit on the Tuesday, and everything looked good. I went home that night, slept well, and the following day also had a good day. Kim was back at work, and so on Thursday, six-days after being discharged from hospital, I was puttering around the house by myself. I found myself upstairs in our little farmhouse attic, doing some rummaging around, not straining myself at all, when all of a sudden, I felt a *pop* in my chest. I stood up straight, tried to take a deep breath, and right away felt something was off. There was decreased airflow in my lungs. I began coughing a bit more than usual, and some blood came up. I went downstairs, took a couple of hits of Ventolin, and waited for ten minutes. I then stood up again, tried to take some deep breaths, and found I was not getting enough oxygen. Plus, I was experiencing quite a bit of pain when I tried to breathe in.

With Kim being thirty minutes away at work, I called my mom and told her I needed to go to St. Paul's immediately. I had had another pneumothorax. I then called Kim and asked her to come by the house and pack a bag for me, as I wouldn't be coming home that night. My mom came within minutes, picked me up, and we were off.

Now, this collapse was not as bad as the previous one. I could walk to the car, sit, and have an easy conversation, but I could feel the familiar heaviness in my chest and my right lung once again felt like a rock.

I had called the clinic ahead of time to let them know I was coming, and they said to go and get an X-ray, then come up to the clinic. They didn't have a bed for me but were hoping one would open up that afternoon. I repeated the steps I had taken ten days prior, hobbling from the elevators to the X-ray, struggling to stand, confirming I was heading straight upstairs to see my doctor, and yes, to get a chest tube put in.

I got to the clinic and was put in an exam room as they waited for a bed to open up on the CF ward. I waited a number of hours, and by that time, Kim had come with my overnight bag, my mom had gone home, and my sister, Lynette, arrived to be with us.

At 5:30 p.m., I was moved from the exam room and into a bed. What happened next was rather surreal. I was given a bed and rolled into a room, but this was no private room—turns out I was going to have three roommates for this chest tube procedure. (That's right. They were going to insert the chest tube right there in the four-person room!) Also, the doctor who came to put the chest tube in was the same medical resident who ten days before had done his first chest tube insertion, on me! And no, he had not had the opportunity to practice since then, but here he was all alone getting this thing in again. Because it took so long to get me into the room, by the time he was ready to go, it was time for nursing shift change. Therefore, my visiting sister (who, I remind you, is a critical care nurse) had to glove up and assist him.

But there we were, curtains drawn around us in this four-person room, the resident doctor once again standing over me, hands gripping the long plastic needle, pushing down with all his might trying to puncture my chest cavity, tube bowing out in the middle, until *poof*(!) through the hard muscle and tissue, straight between the ribs for another perfect shot! The release of air out of the chest tube was even more immediate than the previous one, as I felt an incredible release as the lung began to expand at once. The experience of getting to this place was once again difficult, but the feeling of relief was one of pure bliss. At this point, a new thought came into my head, *Is this how it would feel like to wake up from my transplant and take my first breaths with my new lungs?*

With the chest tube stitched in place, follow-up X-ray done, and me now resting in bed, my doctors were not going to take any chances this time. It was going to be a two-week hospital stay, at minimum. During this hospital stay, I began to get a real taste of hospitalization and how life was going to be going forward.

Within our four-person hospital room, I was the youngest by about twenty years. Immediately to my right was a guy in his mid to late forties. He provided the most entertainment. He was a bit of an ornery guy, and he had unfortunately been in hospital with liver issues for quite some time. We would talk through the curtain throughout the day. The most socially dramatic part of the whole stay was his breakup with his girlfriend right there in the hospital room. Over four days, I listened as the relationship began to show signs of stress, disdain, and then the final shout, "Get the hell out of here and don't come back!"

The woman across the aisle from me was an elderly woman who didn't speak any English. Unfortunately, she could not do much for herself, and I never did learn what it was she was hospitalized for. When she wanted someone's attention, or if the nurse wasn't coming fast enough, she would begin to throw her Mah-jong tiles around the room.

And the last patient to make up our little quad-room was a man in his seventies. He had suffered a major stroke and his whole right side was almost paralyzed. He could lift his arm, but he could not speak. Every day, a speech therapist came to visit him and she would work with him for about thirty minutes.

I was by far the most disruptive person in the room. Everyone, of course, had to listen to my groans while getting my chest tube put in during dinner hour—I can't imagine that was appetizing—then hearing me coughing throughout the night, and then physio during the day. I had a constant stream of doctors and other health professionals come visit me, and I had a few visitors. I hope I provided some entertainment to my roommates, but I was probably one of the patients who made it very difficult to share a hospital room, and why most hospitals today are being built with single-occupancy rooms only.

11.
NEW NORMAL
(PART I)

*"I did not dread what I would become, but I needed
to mourn the end of what I had been.
It was like saying goodbye to a place
I had lived in and loved.*

(*At the Will of the Body,* Arthur W. Frank)

THE SPRING OF 2009 ended up being a time of rest, but also one of being stretched in new and unique ways. It was a season of experiential learning as I tried to settle into a "new normal." The previous summer and fall, when we were going through the workup, was a steep learning curve full of research and reading. Now that we were in the thick of the transplant wait, passing the four, five, and six-month anniversaries of being wait-listed, we were now living out the researched learnings of the previous year.

Though the COVID-19 pandemic has made the phrase "new normal" common and maybe even detestable, it helped provide me with a framework to move through the everchanging challenges of life in 2009. The phrase was first introduced to me by a new friend I made through the pre-transplant team, Margaret. About twenty years older than me, like myself, Margaret also has CF and ten years earlier had received a double-lung transplant.

One thing the transplant agency does, if someone who is waiting requests it, is provide you with a support person, someone who has the same underlying health conditions as you and who has already received the same transplant you are waiting for. This is an amazing source of support. To be able to speak with someone who knows and has experienced the exact things I was going through was such an encouraging experience. As the biblical psalm says, "Deep calls out to deep" (Ps 42:7 NIV).

By the time I got connected with Margaret, I had settled into a restless funk. Up until the end of February, when I was discharged after my second lung collapse, I had not had the time or energy to reflect on what it meant for me to wait for a transplant. After being wait-listed, I began finishing up the home IV treatment I was on, and then it was all about looking forward to Christmas and hoping the transplant wouldn't come before then. Right after Christmas, my sole focus was back on my lungs, as I wasn't feeling well. Another two weeks of home IV antibiotics, and then, of course, February was taken up with the two consecutive pneumothoraxes.

Coming out of February, however, I was starting to feel stable for the first time since being wait-listed. My lungs seemed to have a good seal on them, and the chances of another collapse felt somewhat remote. The two weeks of hospitalization and the rest I was able to get while being there had me feeling the best I had in a number of months. With my acute health concerns now relatively under control, my focus became the *experience* of waiting for transplant.

Now that my mind began focusing on the fact that I was truly *waiting*, I felt a growing anxiety that I wouldn't get my transplant in time. In this state of mind, every week, every day, every hour seemed to stretch out and slowly creep by, bringing me closer to the moment, the split second, when my pager would ring out or closer to the moment when my lungs would ultimately fail.

For the first time in my life, I slipped in and out of depression. What I was experiencing, or fearing, was a complete lack of purpose in my waiting. What was the waiting for if the transplant didn't come? What was all this for? I was waiting for a *chance*, for a *very small* chance. Life was completely on hold. I wasn't working, wasn't traveling, wasn't doing anything else my friends were doing—starting businesses, getting promotions, having families—I was *waiting*. This was my new plot in life, to simply sit and wait.

To sit and wait for anything—a delayed bus, delayed flight, a closed highway—a feeling of absolute helplessness and frustration can rapidly set in if anything can't be done in the meantime to rectify the situation. A complete lack of purpose and meaning is experienced in that moment, a moment that feels lost forever.

This was my state when I was connected with Margaret. She is an incredibly passionate person whose energy and zest for life is contagious, and is a tireless advocate for organ transplantation and honoring donor families. She has worked as a Zumba instructor, elementary school teacher, and is a race-walker and world traveler. It was Margaret who first introduced me to the idea of discovering my new normal. With compassion and empathy, she told me the time had finally come to say goodbye to my old self, which I had known and loved, the one who was carefree, who worked long hours on the farm, and played ice hockey. It was instead time to get acquainted with my new normal and to accept that my life did have a goal and purpose right now. That purpose was a unique one, different from before, but it was maybe, in fact, the most important one I would ever have—I had to begin preparing, right now, for life *after* transplant!

Big Breath In

Talking with Margaret was like a breath of fresh air, but it was also a much-needed kick in the ass! Like my transplant doctor in our early meetings, she didn't sugarcoat anything. First, she said that now was the time I needed to get down to work, and I had to work hard! She spoke with conviction: The transplant *would* come. I had to have faith, but I also couldn't do anything to make it come any faster than it would; therefore, I had to get down to work and make sure that whenever it did come, whether it be the moment after we hung up the phone or in two years, I would be ready! And as she outlined, being ready meant making sure I was as fit and rested as I could be for my surgery and recovery. Whatever I was able to do on this side of the surgery would pay off in massive rewards on the other side.

The second thing she said was that I had to be vigilant in taking care of myself, both now and after transplant. After transplant, I was going to have to learn how to evaluate every situation I was in. Whether that be gardening or in crowded places, evaluating the risk to my new lungs and the likelihood of getting sick wherever I was. Everything in my life had to be seen through the lens of my new lungs; therefore, I had better get started on that now.

It was time to say my goodbyes to those things I knew I couldn't do after transplant, to put to bed any remaining dream of once again dairy farming, and to accept and say goodbye to living carefree in whatever environment I wanted to. It was time to say goodbye to the days when I could leave the house unprepared for what the day would bring. It was time to say goodbye to not worrying about the time because after transplant, the timing of medications was crucial. And it was time to say goodbye to leaving the house without hand sanitizer!

Third, she said it was also time to say goodbye to the image of who I was and to embrace those new things that might seem embarrassing but which could also be my new strength. It was time to accept that whenever I went outside the house, I had to be on oxygen! I was using oxygen while I slept and around the house, especially when exercising, but Margaret challenged me about not wearing it outside. "Why not? Who cares?" she said. "George, this is a matter of your health and life. If people look at you, you can then tell them what it is all about, making them more aware of CF and lung transplants. It is a win-win!" It was time to finally throw all embarrassments aside and to be proud of this new normal. To embrace the opportunity for the new life that I was going to be given, and to do everything in my power to ensure I would be healthy and alive long enough to outwait however long it would take to get my transplant. And it was in this vein that Margaret said it was time I began living in the new normal that had, in reality, already taken shape around me.

For me, there was a two-step approach to developing my new normal. The first step included what I have outlined above: it was the process of accepting the loss of many things that were important to me, but which I could no longer do, *and giving myself the space and permission to grieve that loss.* Developing a new normal meant grieving the loss of the dreams, experiences, and hopes of a life I had once known that were now lost. It meant a process of constant evaluation of the changing circumstances I found myself in and knowing that what once had been was now not. It meant allowing myself to feel the hurt of it all and to look into it and accept that there was a death of something there. This experience is not unlike the death of a loved one, for I was saying goodbye to a life I had loved and dreams I had put so much time and energy into.

The second step, however, was one of hope. I found that after grieving what was lost in the "previous life," the second step became one of taking a look at the new landscape I was in, sizing up what life now looked like, and accepting that there was still a role to play and incredible meaning to find. True, it may not be the role I had once wanted, but this was what life was now looking like and the only way to get through it was not in longing for some former life, not in hoping that all would go back to how it was, but in *accepting* that life was not going to be the same, things already had drastically changed. But that didn't mean it couldn't still be great, it couldn't still be meaningful. Instead, *it could actually be better than what it was*. Developing a new normal meant taking an honest inventory of my life, picking up the viable pieces, and beginning to assemble something new that could carry me through this next chapter.

For me, the best way to begin, and the only way I survived the long wait for transplant, especially the long hospitalizations that were to come, was in forming a new routine for my days. A new "liturgical-formation" to help shape me into my new person and help me find new meaning in each day, no matter how small that was.

It is true, at this point, my life was all about waiting. From a utilitarian stand point, I was not providing much of anything to anyone. I was served by everyone around me because I could do so little for myself. But if waiting was going to be my new *vocation*, then I was going to do it in the most intentional way I could. Preparing myself for the transplant that I had to have faith would one day come.

And this was the final thing that Margaret enlightenment me to, which gave me my new purpose in waiting. She challenged me to change the way I was thinking about waiting, that it was not so much a time of just waiting, but a time of *preparation*. The moment I woke up from my transplant surgery, I needed to hit the ground running. The best way to prepare for my transplant recovery was to make sure I went into my surgery in the best form I could (physically, mentally, and spiritually). This period of waiting was not just waiting for an end goal, the day I got my transplant, but it was preparing for the life I would have after my transplant. This was not a pause in life; it was a time of preparing for something so much better; it was a time to be shaped into my new post-transplant self. And so, from that moment on, my new normal became all about preparing to be a transplant *recipient*.

To help with this transition, and to help me process the changing landscape of my life, I began writing. I began trying to put into words the wrestling I was feeling on the inside. I started to allow my pen (or keyboard) to reveal what was happening inside of me and how I was feeling.

May 30, 2009: *I don't really know what I am feeling, but I know I am not happy with how I am feeling—my emotional state and my physical state. Sometimes you get those days when you are in a bad mood, you know you are in a bad mood and you just don't want to get out of it. My lungs have been bumpin' and popping and gurgling for the past week and I can't quite place my finger on what it is. I have to go into the clinic tomorrow for a checkup, so hopefully it will get figured out then.*

Are You Ready?

People have asked me, "How did you know that you were ready for your transplant?" I didn't have much of a response to this question other than that I knew I would die without it. The doors of life were rapidly closing, and this was the only way through.

I don't think anyone can truly know how they will respond when the call comes. Whether your reaction would be one of joy and excitement, or one of fear and anxiety, or more likely a mixture of both, you can't fully know until the pager all of a sudden begins ringing and vibrating on your hip. There is nothing that can replicate the experience of having your pager, or cellphone, go off, knowing in that second that the whole trajectory of your life has changed!

For me, that moment came on a Thursday morning in May 2009. I had dropped in at my parents' and was now back in my truck, making the five-minute drive home. I had my pager on my right hip, clipped onto my belt as it always was, snuggled between my seat belt and jeans. I was going down the overpass on 112th Street, which crosses over Highway 99. I slowed down and turned right onto Hornby Drive. As I pressed the gas pedal to accelerate back to the speed limit, all of a sudden, into the silence-filled cab of my truck, the heart-stopping, high-pitched beeping of my pager went off! I don't know which sense of mine was activated first, my ears or the touch of the small vibrating black box, but in the millisecond it took to realize what had pierced this mundane Thursday morning, a feeling of pure joy and overwhelming gratitude washed over me. I instinctively let out a howl of excitement and slammed my foot down on the accelerator even harder. *This is it*, I thought. *This is the moment, the second, the series of seconds which will change my life forever!*

I was about two minutes from home and decided I wanted to soak in every moment I was experiencing. I wanted to get home, sit in my truck in our gravel driveway, call the transplant center, and tell them I had heard their beckoning call loud and clear and I was ready. I came through the S-turns on Hornby Drive at top speed and headed down the straightaway to the final turn. I slowed down, made the 90-degree turn onto 104th Street, and punched the gas pedal again as I now only had a kilometer to go before I was home. I couldn't wait any longer. I fished my cell phone out of my left pocket, as I wanted to be ready the moment the truck came to a stop in the driveway and I could hit the call button. I flipped my phone open (yes, this was the days of flip phones) and looked at the time and date. I wanted these to be permanently etched in my mind: 11:04 a.m., *Thursday* . . . *Thursday* . . . *Thursday* . . . *Thursday.* I took my foot off the accelerator, snapped the phone shut, and let it drop to my lap. I coasted the final 200 meters into our driveway, stopped the truck, put it in park, and sat there. *It was Thursday morning.* Thursday morning, or every second Thursday morning, was the day the transplant office tested the pagers. 11:00 a.m. Thursday morning was my test time. I had forgotten it was Thursday morning.

I picked up my phone while still sitting in my truck, called the number on the pager, and said, "Yes, I got the test page. Talk to you again in two weeks. Thanks." It wasn't the most devastating thing I would experience during my wait for transplant, but it was difficult. After recovering from the initial disappointment, I found, however, I was actually grateful for the experience. As I said earlier, people often asked how I knew I was ready for my transplant—this was how I knew. As difficult as the emotional roller coaster of those few minutes was, it showed me, without a shadow of a doubt, that I was ready. I was not only ready, but I *wanted* this with all my heart, soul, and mind. I knew then that when that call eventually came, there would be no hesitation on my part, only pure excitement and gratitude.

Six Months

There was another significant milestone during these spring months. It was a moment of disorientation and grief, which led us once again to an ever-deepening desire for my transplant to come. This event was my six-month anniversary of being wait-listed: May 26, 2009.

The day went by like most other days during that time. Kim went to work, and I went to my own work: physiotherapy. It had now been exactly two months since I was discharged from St. Paul's after the second pneumothorax, and I knew I was slipping again.

I was doing physio three times a day: an hour in the morning, thirty minutes after lunch, and then another hour in the evening. I went for a slow walk outside that day and also visited my parents for lunch. But it was after dinner, sitting at the table with Kim, the dishes having been cleared away, that we began talking about the fact that it had now been a full six months of waiting. So far, I had not been that emotional at all, other than during my lung collapse. But this was the first time the emotions of waiting, the stress that my transplant doctor had talked about the first time we met, finally came bubbling to the surface and pouring out as I held my head in my hands and began sobbing.

I felt the full weight of this waiting reality, of this craving-my-transplant-to-come-but-it-not-coming-yet reality. I felt six months was a long time to be waiting to either die or be given a second chance at life. The heaviness of my life, the stress and angst of waiting for the pager to go off at any second, finally became too much.

May 27, 2009: *It has now been over six months that I have been waiting for my transplant. This past week has been very hard. I don't know if it is because I am not feeling well or if it also has something to do with the fact that it has now been six months. I don't think I properly prepared myself at the beginning of all this to actually wait this long. Even now I find it hard to admit that I might still have to wait a year or more. I know it can easily be that way, but for some reason, I can't actually bring myself to accept that. It could be because I am scared that I don't even have that time left with these lungs. Things have gone downhill so quick that I don't know what* it is like to live in this state. *Everything seems like this could be the end for me, and really, from what the doctors say, I know that I don't have much reserve left and things can get quite bad, quite quickly. And so, it is hard to picture having to wait one or two years for the transplant because right now I can't even picture what my life would look like in a year from now if I don't have the transplant. Will I be able to just keep poking along like this? I don't know.*

The truth is you never know what an experience is like until you go through it yourself. My doctors warned and prepared me as best they could. They had seen many people go through it, but they still could not prepare me for the experience itself. I would talk to other transplant recipients, they could walk alongside me in my struggle, they could share their experience, and that could be a massive comfort and encouragement, but it still could not fully prepare me for the experience of actually living the journey. It is a journey that can only be experienced alone. Even Kim—the closest person in my life, who observed every intimate detail of what I was going through—could not fully share the experience, as her experience was that of a caregiver, close but still not the same.

This was all new for me. In retrospect, I could have prepared myself better. I could have tried harder to enter and imagine the experience of waiting, but it was also such a rare and surreal thing that I could never know it other than by living it. As I wrote back then, even in the middle of waiting, on my sixth-month anniversary, I still could not even imagine what life would look and feel like in a year from then, or even another six months. So much had happened in the previous half-year, so much change, so many new experiences, and such a drastic new normal that I had to grieve and accept. My old life was gone, and trying to look ahead seemed almost impossible.

And yet, I knew I had to continue on. I allowed myself that night, May 26, 2009, the six-month mark of my waiting, to fully look into the grief and loss and experience the weight and stress of it all—to let my emotions run wild and to cry it out. To be present in all the shit-mess that life now was. To accept it and say to myself, *Yes, this is life. It is not the life I want, but it is the life I have to live. And I will live it now because there is hope. Hope of a second chance. Hope of a new life. Hope that one day this weakness will turn into a new strength.* The rest of the evening was fairly subdued. I did my 60 minutes of evening physio before bed, and then Kim and I watched episodes of *Lost* on DVD.

Joy in the Small Things

There is one final note on this transitional season in the spring of 2009. It sounds cliché, but it was the main thing that brought us some unexpected joy. It was the slowing down of life and, for the first time, noticing and taking joy in the small, natural things happening all around us all the time.

I have always loved sunrises and sunsets, and during this time, I found an overwhelming joy in these daily rhythms. Watching the beauty of the sun rise or set over the vast farmland surrounding our little house, I felt I was living the final monologue of Lester Burnham in the movie, *American Beauty*: "Sometimes I feel like I'm seeing it all at once and it's too much. My heart fills up like a balloon that's about to burst. And then I remember to relax and stop trying to hold on to it. And then it flows through me like rain, and I can't feel anything but gratitude for every single moment of my stupid little life."

New Normal (Part I)

It felt like my life was stupid and ridiculous at times, but in these moments of taking in the ineffable beauty of the nature around us, it felt like all the concerns were momentarily suspended.

Early June 2009: *There are a few things that I have noticed lately that I have come to enjoy. It seems that this waiting and slowing down of life are starting to have some effect on me. I have started to become a little calmer in some areas of life. Mainly because I really am in no hurry to get somewhere, until of course my pager goes off. But I have come to take comfort in the small things of life. I love listening to the little things that usually one would not listen to. I found myself smiling at the voice of an old man yesterday. Just the way that most old men talk. Their voices all have a rhythm of breathing that amuses me. That is what I mean, the real small things in life, but it is the things that we all have in common. . . . Everyone has their own story and everyone is an individual, and yet we are so similar.*

July 28, 2009: *Last night we had the biggest thunderstorm in recent memory. As the downpour was happening I opened the front door to watch. As I watched the rain pelt the road, I thought about those scenes in movies and books about India, where the kids go running and playing in the streets when the first rains of the monsoon season hit. Then I thought, I want to go and stand and play in the rain. After all, how often can you stand in the rain around here and not get cold. But then I remembered that I still have my PICC line in that I can't get wet, and I was about to do my physio, so any sort of walking or slight running would just result in a lung hacking fest. Can you imagine me standing in the middle of 104th Street in the middle of a thunderstorm, a garbage bag wrapped around my arm, bent over and hacking up a lung? Kim would probably have to come and save me. It wouldn't be a good sight.*

The spring of 2009 was not so much a series of firsts, but it was a time of coming to grips with what life now looked like. It was a time of grieving the losses we had experienced and accepting the disorientation our life had been thrown into, but also transitioning to a new normal of what a *waiting/preparing life* could look like.

From being listed in November 2008 up to my eventual transplant in 2010, the whole transplant process was a never-ending journey of reorientation—accepting the reality that kept closing in around us and seeking to find some sense of peace and joy in the life we had. I finally allowed my emotions to flow freely during that time, as I didn't have the space inside of me to store them up anymore.

It was also during this time that Kim and I made another big change in our life. Up until this time, we had both been very private people. However, we also knew we had a big community around us. Literally, hundreds of people knew what we were going through, and everyone wanted to know how I was doing. So, we decided to go public. What was happening was that our families were getting inundated with questions as to how I was doing, and every time something happened, I was having to update too many people on what was going on. Soon we found we were stressed out for our families and the barrage of questions they were getting, but also stressed out from having to repeat ourselves to so many people. So, I decided to start a blog. Something that anyone could read to see how I was doing. I was a bit spotty with my entries, but I tried to update as much as I could when I felt well enough to do so. As I look back now, I can see that in the spring and summer of 2009, the seeds of this book were already being planted.

12.
NEW NORMAL
(PART II)

"Our sense of agency, how much we feel in control, is defined by our relationship to our bodies and its rhythms . . . In order to find our voice, we have to be in *our bodies— able to breathe fully and able to access our inner sensations.*
(*The Body Keeps Score,* Bessel Van Der Kolk, MD)

THE REORIENTATION TO a disorientated life proved difficult. Though we were now seeing life through a new lens, knowing that I was going to need IV antibiotics and hospitalizations to try to keep as healthy as possible, it was still a difficult transition to live into. We were still living in the hope that a tune-up of antibiotics could send me sailing into a healthy stretch of time, maybe a month or two, before I would need more help in beating back the killer infections ravishing my airways.

We tried home IV antibiotics once again in June. They started on June 2, five days after my six-month wait-list anniversary. As I

Big Breath In

had experienced before, the routine of appointments I needed to ensure everything went well on home IV antibiotics—PICC line insertion, X-ray, blood work, dressing change, more blood work, PICC line taken out, not to mention the six times a day I would need to hook myself up to the IV pole to get my meds—once again turned out to be exhausting. My body was not able to get the proper rest it needed. After ending the round of antibiotics in mid-June, I lasted only thirteen days until I found myself admitted to hospital for another hit of drugs.

I was admitted to St. Paul's on June 30 and was in hospital for a full two weeks and then discharged for another week of home IV antibiotics, finally finishing up on July 22. This was the first time I had three full weeks of treatment, but it was not going to be the last. In fact, this was now going to be the norm when fighting an infection—a full three weeks of antibiotics—as the usual two-week regimen was not doing the trick. We were slowly finding out a new "George-specific" paradigm of treatment, as I wrote about in a blog post from the day I finished my first three-week stint.

July 22, 2009: *Well I finished my IV antibiotics today. I am glad to be done them, as long as they have worked! I do feel good right now. I am back to my old workout level and my appetite is good . . . let me clarify, by exercise I mean a slow walk on the treadmill using oxygen and then some leg exercises using no weights, just my body weight. So, to a normal person, this is not exercising at all, it is not even considered effort, but for me it will knock me out for the rest of the day. But I do enjoy it!*

As July wound down, my fear of slipping back into active infection once again returned. We were hit with a heat wave right at the end of the month, and it took a devastating toll on my health. The heat wave pushed the temperatures to the mid-thirties (which is very hot for where we live), and life was beginning to feel unbearable. With the heat and the way I was feeling, I also began dealing with anxiety, getting panic attacks as I felt I was not able to catch my breath at times. I tried to sit as still as I could in our house, which was right on the ocean, and allow the breeze to blow through the windows, but all I could feel was the sweat trickling down my face, my shirt getting wet with perspiration, and mucus welling up in my airways while I tried to suppress the act of coughing so as not to push my body temperature to what felt like a breaking point. On July 30, I took to my blog.

July 30, 2009: *Many of you have been asking how I am doing with the heat, and I really appreciate your concern because I am having quite a hard time with it. It already takes a lot of energy to breathe, and now with the heat, it causes me to get real hot real fast, not to mention that I am not getting much rest, because like everyone, I don't sleep well in the heat. With being so run down, my CF symptoms spring to life, compounding my regular struggles, and are making life very uncomfortable and at times worrisome. I spent yesterday at my uncle and aunt's place in their air-conditioned basement, so that brought some much-needed relief, but as soon as I got home, things got quite unbearable until about 10:30 p.m. when the ocean tide began to come in and there was a slight breeze coming off the bay. . . I will have to wait and see if I will be able to recover from the stress that the heat put on my body, and the subsequent symptoms I have developed again. At this time, I am in this constant cycle of feeling run down, which is starting to take its toll.*

Five days later, I was admitted to hospital. Usually, when a person with CF is admitted to hospital, they are able to coordinate with the CF clinic and wait at home until a bed is ready so that they can be admitted straight to the CF ward and forgo the usual wait in

Big Breath In

the admissions department. This time, I couldn't wait. I had been in contact with the CF clinic for a day and a half, but I wasn't the only one struggling in the heat—there were no CF beds opening up as everyone was suffering. Finally, I called them again on the second afternoon of knowing I needed to come in, told them how I was doing, and their reply was that I needed to come into hospital right away. I was told to go straight to the ER, as this would be the fastest way to get the much-needed antibiotics started. This was one of the worst admitting experiences I had, as I wrote in my blog upon discharge from hospital three weeks later.

I was feeling VERY sick at the time of admission. I was having trouble walking even a couple steps while on oxygen, so we knew I had to be admitted. Because it was a very quick admission, basically an emergency, I was put in the only bed they had (on the CF floor), which was in a four-bed public room. Usually they try to get the CF patients into private rooms for infection control reasons, but all they had was the public room, which I was okay with because all I wanted to do was lie down and get those antibiotics started. But no sooner than my first big coughing fit did I realize that it wasn't me who was most upset about being in this room; it was the other three patients, all of whom were over sixty and who didn't have any sort of respiratory problems. I awoke from a nap on my second day to hear a nurse explaining to the elderly woman across from me that, "Just as you can't catch asthma from someone else, you can't catch CF either." I had to smile. Throughout those first 48 hours my nurses would come by and update me on the room situation and when I would be moving to a private room. Through the curtain I would also hear my neighbors whispering to their visitors when they would quietly inquire about "that guy" behind the curtain doing all the coughing. After two days, I was transferred to a private room; I was not the only one who was relieved I was being moved!

It took three days to feel that the antibiotics were kicking in and providing some relief. When I finally landed in a private room, I was able to come off oxygen for periods of time during the day, although it wasn't until a full week passed that I could exercise again on the treadmill. From this time on, during hospitalizations, it usually took a good four to seven days before I would have the energy and breathing capacity to exercise, and each time, it was like starting from scratch with atrophied leg muscles from lying and sitting around for more than a week.

New Normal = New Routines

When I began feeling better during this hospital admission, I began settling into some new rhythms and routines while in hospital. For me, to survive these longer stints in hospital meant having a routine that I could follow almost every day.

I would usually wake up and get out of bed around 7:45 a.m. I'd go to the bathroom, then sit on the edge of my bed with my kidney tray (a small kidney shaped plastic bowl), and begin coughing. I would usually sit for about five minutes, coughing up all the mucus that had accumulated in my lungs overnight, or at least since I last woke up during the night to do the same.

I would get this first fit of coughing out of the way, empty my kidney tray of mucus, and be back on the side of my bed, watching the morning news by the time my breakfast arrived, usually around 8:00 a.m. Oatmeal, eggs, two pieces of toast, two milks, and a cup of tea was my standard breakfast.

I would polish this off in about fifteen minutes and then, around 8:30 a.m., would dive into my first round of physiotherapy. By now, my nurse would have come in and delivered all my physio meds, hooked me up for a round of IV antibiotics, and taken a set of vitals (heart rate, blood pressure, temperature, O2 stats). My physio would last for about 60 to 90 minutes, depending on what kind of new meds I was put on (inhaled antibiotics) and how much coughing there would be and how long it would take to catch my breath. Then, usually around 10:00 a.m., my physiotherapist would come and take me over to the CF gym for about 45 minutes of light exercise on the treadmill or rowing machine.

Getting back to my room around 11:00 a.m., I would pick up a couple towels from the housekeeping cart in the hallways, make sure my oxygen line wasn't wrapped around anything in my room and that it would reach comfortably into my bathroom, and then strip down and have a nice hot shower. I would put on a new shirt each day while wearing the same PJ pants for a couple of days in a row. By this time, lunch would usually be waiting for me on the tray table. I would often watch the TV show *King of Queens* while eating lunch. After this, I'd begin my second round of physio, usually lasting about 45 minutes.

In the afternoon, I would either continue watching TV, lie back in my bed, and listen to music, or, if I was feeling *really* good, attempt to read something. But most often, I took an afternoon nap. With all the noise of a hospital, both during the day and at night, I always tried to sneak some naps in wherever I could get them, as sleep was a precious commodity. Of course, throughout this whole time, I would be getting hooked and unhooked from my IV pole as I was on two different antibiotics, one of them being every six hours and the other every four.

The most boring time of the day was between 3:30 and 5:00 p.m., when there was nothing on TV, and I was too fatigued to do much else but lie in my bed. At 5:00 p.m., I would turn on the news, which would provide some distraction, and begin looking forward to dinner, which would arrive at 6:00 p.m. Between 5:00 and 5:30 p.m., Kim would arrive with a duffle bag full of washed clothes or more snacks and other miscellaneous supplies. After dropping this off, she then often walked back down to the street to buy me a burger and fries, fattening food that was dearly needed.

Then, 7:00 p.m. would bring shift change for the nurses, my evening physio meds, and being hooked back up to my IV pole for the night. My evening physio would take about an hour. Usually, Kim would leave between 8:00 and 8:30 p.m., after we finished watching whatever show we were into at the time on our portable DVD player. I would then usually watch some TV on my own until around 9:30, which is when I would begin packing it in for the day, cleaning up my room a bit, brushing my teeth, and getting under the covers by 10:00 p.m.

These were long days, but keeping to this routine helped meld the days together to make them seem not so long. Also, keeping to a regimented routine helped give me something to do, a schedule to follow, and even a bit of a purpose and a goal to complete—a sense of accomplishment, no matter how small it was. When so much control in life is lost, this schedule and routine was something that was still mine. It helped provide some controllable structure. It would often be interrupted by nurses, doctors, or other medical professionals throughout the day, but it was a structure that helped orientate the long days in hospital. Everyone is different, but being who I am, this daily routine turned out to be crucial to my emotional and mental health during this time of disorientation and disempowerment.

But of course, after the two, then three, and later, many more weeks of living in the hospital, nothing beat coming home and being able to throw this routine out the window in order to just relax. As I wrote the day after being discharged on August 26: *It is so nice to wake up this morning to the sound of Kim getting out of bed rather than the lab tech coming to draw more blood.*

That day, however, also marked nine months of waiting for my transplant.

August 26, 2009: *I have gained a new respect for expecting mothers, as I never really realized how long nine-months can be, especially when waiting for something exciting and life changing. Upon further reflection, I began to draw some similarities between my wait for a transplant and a pregnant mother's wait for their coming child. I couldn't sleep the last night that I was in the hospital, so I came up with a list of parallels. Upon further reflection the next morning, the cleverness from the night before didn't seem so clever in the light of day, so I scratched the list. But what I will leave you with are two thoughts and parallels that exist between waiting for lungs and waiting for a baby: just as the first scream from a newborn baby symbolizes its first deep breath of air, so too will the scream of my pager symbolize and set in motion events that will lead to what will feel like my first deep breath of air. And second, with pregnancy and with transplantation may come anxiety, worry, and a lot of waiting, but all of that will be outweighed by the joy that the coming gift will bring.*

Transplant FAQs

The three-week hospital stay in August ended up doing wonders for my health. Though it had been a tough summer, the cocktail of antibiotics my doctors had got me on finally seemed to do the trick. I was able to stay out of hospital for a little over three months after that, the longest I would be out of hospital until my eventual transplant.

As August turned into September, Kim and I attended the wedding of one of my cousins. It felt good to be relatively well enough to get out and see people. Though we didn't light up the dance floor or walk around much (Kim had to bring me my food from the buffet table), it was refreshing to be in a social setting again, even with my oxygen tank trailing behind me.

This was the first time my extended family had seen me since being wait-listed nine months earlier; therefore, there was a lot to talk about and a lot of questions that came out.

1. *How many people are on the wait list and where are you on it?* At that time, there were fifteen people waiting for a single lung transplant, and another six of us waiting for a double.

2. *What is the average wait time for a double-lung transplant?* When I was wait-listed, I was told the average wait time for a double-lung transplant was eight months; however, during the time I was waiting, BC was going through a dry spell. In the previous twelve months, only two double-lung transplants had been done, whereas they usually did an average five in a year. (Note: Today, in 2021, the wait time in BC has improved dramatically, often measured in weeks rather than months. This is due to increased awareness of organ transplants, but also, tragically, because of an increase in donors due to the opioid-overdose crisis gripping our province.)

3. *Where I was on the wait list?* That was always very difficult to answer. The decision of who gets the lungs that became available is made by the head transplant doctor, along with the surgeon, and it was usually based on most need and best match. I don't know how it works today, but back in the day, my transplant doctor carried a list

with all the names and medical info of all the wait-listed people. This way, no matter where he was, when he got a call from any hospital in BC telling him they have a lung or set of lungs available for transplant, he would need to decide who would get them and then pass that info to the on-call coordinator.

4. *What happens when the call comes?* Once the call comes, I would have to call the transplant center and get instructions. But 30% of all transplant calls are false alarms (remember that!). This means that everything looks good on paper, but once the surgeon takes the lungs out of the donor, they may find a problem that prevents them from going ahead with the transplant; this problem is usually damage done to the lungs while they are trying to coordinate the transplant. However, they want you to come to the hospital right away. At the hospital, they will do an X-ray and lots of blood tests. The surgery can still be called off even when the patient is in the OR, ready to be put under. This is obviously very discouraging and the hardest part of the process, if it happens.

5. *What about the surgery and recovery?* If the donor lungs are good and the transplant goes ahead, the surgery would take between eight to ten hours. You then go to the ICU for a number of days, if not a week or more, and then the transplant ward, often for a few more weeks. The time that each patient spends in the ICU and on the ward is different since every patient experiences different setbacks. One thing that seems to be common from the stories I heard is that everyone suffers some sort of setback after surgery;

therefore, we were told to expect it and not be anxious when/if it happens.

The Merging of Tragedy and Hope

My cousin's wedding and the weeks that followed were my final season of levity before my transplant. Whereas the summer had been tough, battling a stubborn lung infection that would not come under control, the fall of 2009 was a time of stable health. It was a season in which we finally settled into living life day-by-day and not looking too far into the future. Kim got a pretty bad cold near the end of September, which had us walking on eggshells for the better part of two weeks, wondering if I would get it and thus have to report back to the hospital, but somehow, I was able to keep clear of it.

After trying to develop a new normal throughout the spring and summer of that year, this fall season turned into a deeper time of reflection. Around this time, I was growing aware of tension building up inside of me. We were now at a place where Kim and I, our families, and everyone in our larger community was longing for me to get this transplant. As a family, it seemed we had one central focus: getting my transplant. Yet, the awareness that what we were waiting for was someone else to die in such a way that I could receive their lungs was becoming more troublesome for me. I ended up speaking with my social worker a number of times about this issue, as I was having a hard time separating my potential donor's death from my opportunity at life. Over time, however, I was able to begin to separate the two a bit. For me, my donor's eventual death and my eventual transplant were emotionally tied up into one event. I couldn't separate the two events; it was as if my waiting begat their death. But in talking with my social worker and others, I began to see that the death of my potential donor and me receiving a transplant were actually unrelated events. The person who would be my donor was going to die, and they would die whether I was wait-listed and could receive their organs or not. The two events were not related. However, the connection would come from the donor's family. In donating their loved one's organs, donor families often feel that this giving of life through transplant can be a ray of light in someone's tragic death. What is often experienced by donor families, though grieving as they are, is that transplantation can often provide them some sense of purpose, or at least ease their sorrow, however small. My transplant would not be the cause of someone's death, but it could be a sliver of light and meaning to a family's overwhelming grief.

My sister, Lynette—who as an ICU nurse has firsthand experience with both the tragedy of death and the hope of new life that is involved in the transplant process—spoke about experiences of donor families that she had witnessed countless times. In a keynote address she delivered at a critical care conference a couple of years after my transplant, she said: "For families who know their loved one's wishes regarding donation, it can provide hope in what we all know to be a hopeless situation. I have seen families cling to the hope that someone else may benefit from what so often seems like a senseless death. I have also seen the heartache of a family desperately wanting to be able to donate their loved one's organs in a situation where they were not candidates. Looking for something good, looking for some meaning, for sense in their tragic loss. Organ donation goes far beyond the exchange of one organ for another."

There was nothing we could do as a family to speed the transplant process along. We were simply waiting, but I suppose this is a good thing. For what we were really doing was waiting for this merging of families, a merging of experiences and emotions:

of deep grief and heartfelt gratitude, of final goodbyes and hope for a new future. Organ transplantation is not only a moving of organs from one person to another, but it is a sharing and passing on of life.

What to Say

As I was getting sicker, and as we were waiting longer and longer, we got a lot of offers for help. The truth was, though, there was not that much that people could do for us. There isn't a lot to do when you are spending a lot of time in hospital or sitting around the house. However, in addition to offers for help, some of the more sensitive people would ask, "What can people *say* that is helpful or appreciated?" This is an excellent question! Suffering, waiting, and depression are already incredibly difficult experiences to go through, but these experiences can often be made worse by people's comments. People often mean well, but sometimes, when the listener is in a vulnerable state, comments can sound insensitive and often cause more hurt or drive the dagger of suffering even deeper.

I have come to learn that platitude and clichés do nothing to help anyone, and often the best thing one can do is somehow signal to the sick or suffering person that they are being heard and seen. The best way to do this is to feed back to them what you are hearing and affirm the emotions and experiences being shared. People who are hurting, who are not living the life they want because of either physical or mental illness, don't need to hear that "Everything will be okay" or "God has a plan." These sentiments can often be offensive. What they most often need is a verbal or nonverbal affirmation that what they are going through has been seen and, in that, validated. They want to know that you as family or friend are *bearing witness* to their hurt, seeing the difficult emotions, and even naming the *unknowingness* of what they are going through.

Megan Devine, in her book, *It's Okay That You're Not Okay*, writes, "To truly feel comforted by someone, you need to feel heard in your pain. You need the reality of your loss reflected back to you—not diminished, not diluted. It seems counterintuitive, but true comfort in grief is in acknowledging the pain, not in trying to make it go away."

What was most supportive during my wait was the presence of a listening ear when I felt like talking and, at other times, someone who would sit in the silence, not say anything but just be physically present. I enjoyed getting emails, letters, and cards, as I could reread these as needed, or toss them if they missed the mark. I also enjoyed hearing about other people's lives. I didn't enjoy their complaining (don't ever complain about your life when sitting with someone suffering in a hospital), but I liked hearing about the everyday mundane things my friends were experiencing—what their commute was like, what they were working on at their job, and how their kids were doing in school. Since I wasn't getting out much and I didn't see many people, so much of my life was solely focused on me, thus I found it enjoyable to hear about other people's lives (in moderation). I wasn't looking for anything magical or uplifting, just something genuine.

Counting Down to a Year

There were a couple of significant milestones that passed during the fall of 2009. In September and October, I passed the ten- and eleven-month mark of waiting for transplant. During these milestones, I realized, how fast time was actually moving. If you had told me at the beginning of the transplant journey, or even just a couple month before, that I would have to wait eleven months, that would have been an overwhelming prospect. But time kept ticking by, and slowly but surely, we marked its passing.

At the end of September, I remember remarking how it felt like we were entering the "red zone." Most of the transplant recipients I had been in contact with or had heard about had got their transplant between months ten and fourteen. Therefore, as we passed the ten-month mark, the stakes seemed to get a bit higher. As real as the waiting and whole experience was before this, it now ratcheting up even more!

These stakes raised even higher when, on October 26, the eleven-month anniversary of being wait-listed, Kim and I had a clinic visit with my transplant doctor and I was informed that I was being moved to the "high-priority" list. This would mean that for people of my size and blood type, I was now at the front of the line, which also meant I was the sickest person on the list. This move to high-priority was mainly due to the difficulty I had over the summer in bringing the infections in my lungs under control, the continued small bleeds I was having, and simply the amount of time I had been waiting. Mostly though, it symbolized that things were not going to be getting any better anytime soon and now was the optimal time for transplant. My CF doctor echoed these sentiments when, around this same time, having to hold my medical chart with two hands because of its bulging size, commented, "Having a file this big means it is time to get this transplant done!"

We were grateful and excited about this move to the top of the list. At the time I was waitlisted, I was able to estimate how many people were ahead of me. As I mentioned earlier, BC was going through a dry spell in terms of lung transplants, and so it was getting quite depressing to think that with transplant being so rare, and with a number of people still ahead of me on the list, getting mine was going to take forever, if it ever came at all. Yes, being given high priority meant I was very sick and getting closer to death, but at least, I knew I had a good shot at getting any lungs that became available and were the right match for me.

As October turned to November, and I had been at home and off IV antibiotics for over two months, the stress lines in my health once again began to show. Each day seemed to present something different from the last. One day, I would feel fine; the next day, I would have my phone in my hand, ready to call the CF clinic, and then the following day, I would feel relief again. Sometimes my symptoms would fluctuate between morning and afternoon, almost hour by hour!

The past two weeks have been frustrating. I seem to have a couple good days then a bunch of bad days, then a couple good day and then more bad ones. My body seems to have a battle going on inside of it. I have felt myself going downhill this past week. I feel fine in the mornings, but by the evening, I am feeling very tired and quite short of breath. Also, Wednesday and Thursday night I could not fall asleep, which is usually a sign of bad things to come. Yesterday, I was very tired and ready to wave the white flag, but then I fell asleep just fine, and this morning, I woke up feeling better, but now my lungs are starting to show symptoms again. So, if you ask me how I am doing right now I would have to say, "I don't know. I just can't get a clear read."

And that was how it often was during this season of waiting. I often didn't even know how I was feeling, and one of the most demoralizing things was not being able to get a read on how I was feeling because it was changing so quickly.

New Normal (Part II)

For the most part I felt quite good this weekend. It is like I wrote a couple weeks ago: symptoms seem to come and go making it hard to get a handle on things. I am not as tired and short of breath as last week, but now my lungs are doing different things that are kind of hard to explain. So, it is still the same old thing, one day at a time.

At a CF clinic visit on November 10, my CF doctors said it was probably time for a tune-up. Better to do this now—have me admitted for antibiotics when things were still relatively stable, rather than wait for it to get out of control. I was able to wait at home for a couple of days for a bed and private room to open up. I went in for two weeks of antibiotics. My body responded well, and after two weeks, I was discharged to finish up my final week of antibiotics at home.

During this week of home antibiotics, we marked the one-year anniversary of being wait-listed. It was a strange feeling, a day of pride that I had made it this far and waited this long, but also a depressing day, as it represented the helpless state we found ourselves in, of wanting this so bad but having no control over it.

November 26, 2009: *One year; twelve months; fifty-two weeks; three hundred and sixty-five days: Call it what you will, but as of 2:30 p.m. today, I will have officially been waiting one year for my transplant. I am able to see today as a bit of a milestone. I am very thankful and glad that I am feeling half decent today as I am still on IV antibiotics, because I know that if I was feeling crappy then today would be more depressing. To be totally honest, I never thought I would be waiting this long. I know the doctors said that some people do have to wait even two years, but when I was put on the transplant list, there were only four of us on there, and the last couple years, they have been doing five or six double-lung transplants every year. But this has been a very slow year for lung transplants. And so, we* *will continue to wait. I am very thankful that I was listed when I was. Each day that passes is another day closer to transplant. I am very excited for the transplant. I think I am about 99% excited and 1% anxious, you can never get rid of all the anxiety. I know the transplant can still be a long way off, and so we will continue to live one day at a time, but today is special, and it is a milestone.*

13.
SILENT NIGHT

"Hallelujah, holy shit!"
(National Lampoon's Christmas Vacation,
Clark Griswold)

DECEMBER 2009 WAS another difficult season in our transplant journey. In November, I had already spent two weeks in hospital, being discharged for my final week of antibiotics at home. It had taken a couple of days to feel the effects of the drugs, but they seemed to be doing something by the time we finished the first week of meds, and from there, it seemed to keep improving. Feeling pretty strong after the two weeks, I went home to finish up my meds, which was a good week, being able to make some small improvements at home.

However, within days of coming off the antibiotics, I could tell the drugs I was on didn't get the best kill possible. It was as if the bacteria, knowing the onslaught of antibiotic bombing was coming, retreated and gave up ground quickly so they could go deep and hide until the attack was over, to be ready to emerge back into the major airways once the meds were done. Five days after coming off antibiotics, I called the clinic and told them, "I think

I need to come in again." The following day, they had a bed ready and I was back in the big house.

Just as the previous summer had been a battle that saw three back-to-back admissions, my doctors saw it was time to make another transition and kiss home IV goodbye for good. I was done with that program, as it just wasn't working, and it was now time to spend three full weeks in hospital. I was admitted on December 10, and though I was not told outright that I would be in hospital over Christmas, my doctors hinted I should begin preparing for this possibility.

During that admission, when my CF doctor came to see how I was doing, they would kick the discharge date a little further down the road each time, never really giving me a definitive answer as to how long I would be in hospital. Doctors usually try their best to get patients out of hospital for Christmas. Like much of life, a lot of stuff in the hospital shuts down, or at least slows down, during the major holidays. After I had been in hospital for about eleven days, bringing us to December 20, my CF doctors finally made the call that I had not yet made enough progress and would be spending Christmas 2009 in hospital.

It is a rather surreal thing, being in hospital over Christmas. Of course, every year, there are thousands of people in hospital over the holidays, but it was a rather depressing scene, especially as I come from a family and tradition that usually makes a pretty big deal of the season and of getting together!

When Christmas Eve and Christmas Day rolled around, I was able to get a day pass to go home. I would receive my noon meds by mid-morning, an hour or two early. Kim would then arrive each day to pick me up. I was allowed to skip my afternoon meds, but then had to be back to get my evening meds by 8:00 p.m.

On Christmas Eve, Kim picked me up at lunchtime and we headed home for a couple of hours. We spent the afternoon together and then went to my parents. Lynette and Bryan were traveling in India that year, so our Christmas celebration was already a bit muted. We had our regular Christmas turkey dinner, which included buttered up massed potatoes, thick gravy, cooked carrots, and, of course, cranberry sauce, all which tasted like heaven after eating hospital food the previous two weeks. The four of us then moved over to the living room for desserts (of course I ate way too many) and exchanging some small gifts. I talked about what it was like to spend the lead-up to Christmas on the ward. The nurses were dressed in Christmas scrubs, a tree was set up at the nursing station, which was just outside my room, and there was usually Christmas music playing in the hallway. (I admit I am a scrooge when it comes to Christmas music, not a fan at all.) It was a good effort the staff were making, and I appreciated everything they were doing to make it feel like a special season, but it could not cover up the fact that the hospital was a rotten place to be on Christmas.

The thing we did not talk about as a family—but which seemed to stand as a pink elephant in the middle of the room, seemingly tottering from side to side, threatening to crush us all under its weight—was the feeling that if the following year was anything like the previous one, then this would probably be my last Christmas. Either I was going to get my transplant in the coming year, or I would not live to see the end of it.

The previous Christmas, though I was uncomfortable and was waiting to get on antibiotics, we felt full of hope. It had been full of those things that we had always celebrated at this time of year, both as a family and in our church—hope, peace, joy and love. I had been waiting for my transplant for a month, and we were somehow sure that 2009 was going to be a great year, one where I would experience a whole new life in receiving my transplant. We felt assured that as a family we would once again be sitting in my parents living room, having dessert and opening gifts, with me being healthy and all of us sharing stories and giving thanks for the transplant I had received. Now, a year later, constantly watching the clock to see when Kim and I would have to leave to get me back to the hospital, we were all silently wondering if we would ever do this again. Strong was the love that year, but fragile was the hope, peace, and joy.

The following morning, Christmas Day, I woke up to silence. It may have been the one morning when I woke up in hospital, and for a couple of moments, there was not a sound on the ward. Anyone who could have been discharged had been sent home during the previous day or two. It was now just the nurses, one doctor, and the sickest of the sickest patients, those too fragile to sleep at home or miss a dose of treatment.

Once again, Kim came and picked me up late morning, and we spent the rest of the day together in our house. We exchanged some gifts, watched some Christmas movies, and tried to relax, not thinking about the potential dread of the coming year. We usually got together with Kim's family on Christmas Day, but due to me being in hospital and one of her brother's and his wife being out of town, we postponed those celebrations until the new year.

Kim dropped me off at the hospital an hour late that night. I had to hobble over to the emergency department to get back into the hospital, as all the other doors had already been automatically locked. I had to explain to the security guard that I was a patient trying to get back to my room. As I was getting onto the elevators, I got a phone call from my nurse, wondering where I was, as now I was really late for my meds. When I got to the floor, my nurse wasn't too happy with me, but she also smiled and understood. It was a difficult day for everyone in the hospital, patients and staff included.

The hospital began waking up from its Christmas slumber on December 27, with my CF doctors coming to check on how the previous days had gone. Despite my skipped meds on December 24 and 25, I had made some good progress and was feeling better. It looked like three weeks was all I was going to need.

I was discharged on December 30. However, if Christmas Eve had been depressing, New Year's Eve, which is usually a general time of reflection for me, was just as bad, knowing that as the calendar flipped, this was going to be the year that my life would change forever—for good or for bad. I knew that 2010 was going to be a big year. I knew I would not survive another year like I had just gone through. This year was going to be different; we just didn't yet know yet what that difference would be.

14.
THE NARROWING OF LIFE

> "Here, on the borders of death, life follows an amazingly simple course, it is limited to what is most necessary, all else lies buried in gloomy sleep . . .
> As in a polar expedition, every expression of life must serve only the preservation of existence, and is absolutely focused on that."
>
> (*All Quiet on the Western Front,*
> Erich Maria Remarque)

AS WE FLIPPED the calendar from 2009 to 2010, I feared the worst. One of the biggest things this wait for transplant was doing was making me become very aware of time and its ever-passing nature. Ever since the age of eight, I've worn a wristwatch. I always wanted to know what time it was. As I spent more and more days in hospital, my routine became my saving grace for staying sane. It didn't help me forget time, but the regimenting of it through daily rhythms gave me an illusion of some control over it. Knowing how long things took and filling that time with certain activities to make the time pass gave me a certain kind of meaning so it didn't feel like I was just wasting time. But, of course, the paramount question that kept rolling around in my mind was, *How much time is left? How much time is left in my wait for transplant? How much time is left if my transplant never comes?*

Little did I know that as I got up on New Year's Day 2010, this would be the year that the most important moment of my life would take place. It was still a long way off, and there was still a lot of waiting and suffering to go through, but as I look back now, as much as I was yearning for the moment when my pager would go off, I now see just how short those days were.

Something else was happening on January 1, 2010. Someone else was also changing the calendar that year, but was changing it for the final time. At some point in our lives, we will all change our last calendar. We will all one day celebrate our final New Year's. It is a fact of life.

For me, today, in writing these sentences some eleven years since my transplant, eleven years since my donor passed away, it is still hard to fathom how essential this person has been to me, but also how they remain a complete mystery. They are the person who has had the greatest impact on my life but who stands in a complete fog. I know they are there, standing next to me, present within me. Yet they have no idea what they have done for me, the impact their death has had on me and my family, and I have no clue who they are. I hold and seek to steward to the best of my ability the vital part of their body they gave me, and yet, my thanks to them has no object to which it can attach itself.

My donor and I would have entered 2010 in the same geographical region, but I can only guess that our perceptions of the future were very different. Me, conscious of every day slipping past, and he or she, most likely making plans for the year to come.

But with the changing of the calendar, we were both on a journey heading toward a single day where our lives, and the lives of those closest to us, would explode in an emotional outpouring. One of grief, and the other of gratitude.

The beginning of 2010 began an unprecedented time in my life. It was a time in which I would come to feel more comfortable and safe living in hospital than at home. After the Christmas admission of 2009, I was home for a total of nine days before being admitted again to hospital. This, of course, was now my third admissions in two months. It seemed that this was going to be the new cadence of my life. My doctors began hinting that there wasn't much hope of actually killing the bacteria that was ravishing my airways; the antibiotics were now simply holding things at bay. We were at a place with my lung infections where there was no cavalry coming to save the day. We were fighting a losing battle, and the loss was already a forgone conclusion. It was now all about trying to hold the enemy off long enough to be evacuated from this fighting field, and then given a whole new chance on a new and clean field (a new set of lungs). My CF doctors were trying to find the right balance of fighting and rest; applying the right specialized forces (the right antibiotics) at the right time, while holding back the last-ditch efforts (the lethal antibiotics, which would carpet bomb everything in sight, leading to lifelong side effects), but also giving the troops a rest, making sure my kidneys and mental health could get a break every now and then, to get me back home and remind me of what I was fighting for.

I was admitted to hospital on January 8, 2010. The reason for these repeated hospital admissions was because I was developing resistance to many of the drugs I was regularly on. They would knock the infection back but couldn't ever kill it. I cruised through the three weeks in hospital at the beginning of the year by sticking to my regular routine. But for the first time, I found myself having mixed emotions about going home when the three weeks were up. On January 29, 2010, the day I was discharged, I wrote a blog post.

January 29, 2010: *I am a bit apprehensive about being home as I don't know what my health is going to do next, if I will stay well or get sick again. It is good to be out of the hospital though and off IV medication. As far as my health goes, I am not going to say too much. I am stable enough to be at home right now, but that is about it. I don't expect much from my lungs anymore. The doctor said that if I end up back in the hospital soon, it will mean long-term antibiotics, and by long term, he means a couple of months rather than weeks.*

Close Call

There was one interesting note to make of that January 2010 hospital admission. During that stay, my transplant doctor came to see me. He had a train of five interns behind him and asked me a bunch of questions about my health I was sure he already knew the answers to. But he also mentioned that back on Boxing Day, I had a very close call to getting my transplant. He said that they had a set of lungs that would have fit my size and the blood type as a match. In fact, everything on paper was perfect, except that one of the lungs showed signs of damage, and so it was decided at the last minute to change strategies and instead do a single-lung transplant on someone who was waiting for just one lung. He said it was a tough decision to make, but they wanted to give me the best shot possible at two healthy lungs.

There were two ways to react to this news. One was to pout and ask why they didn't just do it and give them to me (surely even with some damage, these new lungs would still give me a better chance than what I was living with right now). But my reaction was actually the opposite. Though my health was very fragile, we were not yet at the point of taking on the risk of lungs that were anything but near perfect. I wrote in my blog at that time: *We are in this for the long haul. I want to be given the best chance I can have for a long and healthy life post-transplant, and the doctors feel the same way. Of course, as I get sicker the standards for quality of lungs will come down, simply because at some point we will have to get this done. But I am glad to see that the doctors are not in desperation mode yet.*

A Very Fine Line

After being released from hospital at the end of January, we got an unexpected surprise as I was able to be home for a full month, which was perfect because this was the exact time the Vancouver 2010 Olympics were happening. Over the following month, I would spend all my time sleeping, eating, doing physio, and watching Canada kick some Olympic ass! On the health side of things, every day seemed to be about walking the very fine line between being at home and having to go back into hospital. Because of the Olympics, the hospital was encouraging the different clinics, that if their patients were healthy enough, to have them be at home. The downtown core of the city did not need any more people driving there, and because of the events in the city, they were trying to keep the hospitals as empty as possible in case of any large-scale security emergency. Some blog posts from the time speak to the tightrope I often felt I was walking.

February 7, 2010: *I have wanted to write over the past couple days, but it has been difficult to know how I am actually doing. Things are* *very up and down right now. I will be feeling comfortable and then five minutes later, I will begin to feel fatigued and all of a sudden my mucus production will gone into "flow mode," where it feels like a constant flow of mucus coming from my lungs. I am not sleeping well either, but I guess I am keeping my head above water.*

February 12, 2010: *I suppose the best way to describe how I am doing is that I am just kind of standing still: not getting much better, but not getting much worse. Time just keeps on going and the days continue to pass and I am still at home, so that at least is a good thing. I am on an inhaled antibiotic right now which I think has helped.*

February 19, 2010: *Well I have now been home for three weeks, which has been nice. It is still a fine line between being home and knowing when to go into the hospital, but I have been feeling comfortable the last couple days. I am just happy to be off IV antibiotics for a couple weeks to give my body a break.*

At this point, I was doing six hours of physio a day, plus two hours of napping in the afternoon. Trying to survive each day had literally become a full-time job. The only difference was that taking a day off "work" was not an option.

The Fight to Find the Right Cocktail

Out of curiosity, I started doing some calculations. I figured out that in 2009, I had received 82 liters of IV medications. If you added the month of December 2008 to that, it was 99 liters.

When in hospital, I also noticed that the price of each bag of antibiotic was printed on the medication sticker. One antibiotic in particular, which I was on a lot, was only $5 a dose. However, a second drug that I was also on a lot cost $100 a dose, and I received that drug six times a day in hospital. In fact, during my next hospital stay, which is better numbered in months rather than weeks, I received over $100,000 worth of that one drug alone!

March 5, 2010: *I am heading back into St. Paul's today. This past week I have been feeling more and more short of breath. The new inhaled antibiotic does not seem to be working anymore. They don't have a bed for me, so I have to go through emergency, which sucks.*

Thus began the longest hospital stay of my life—a little over two months. We didn't know it at the time, but I would now be what is best phrased as *living in hospital*. There were three factors that lead to such a long admission. First, it was clear that the three-week hospital stints were no longer working. So, from the beginning, we knew this was going to be a long stay. The second factor had to do with recognizing how fragile my health was. My lungs were on their last gasps and didn't have the ability to fight these infections on their own. But the third factor that led to the long admission, which is one of the greatest fears of people living with CF, is we were no longer able to find the right antibiotic cocktail to treat the infections.

    The bacteria inside my lungs were so fortified in the mucus and had developed so much resistance to so many drugs that I had already been on that we were coming down the wire on how to hold them at bay. No matter what the doctors threw at the bacteria, it seemed the bugs already had the armor to withstand the assault. Or if the infection was beat back for a day or two, it found a new way to outflank the antibiotics, adapting itself, and once again showing off its new resistance.

During the nine-week hospital stay, I was tried on five different antibiotics, using six different combinations of those five drugs, and two dosing changes to try to break the bacteria code. All of this ended up bringing me to the brink of being rushed to the intensive care unit because of an all-out allergic reaction in my lungs.

Things started out okay when I was first admitted in early March. I didn't have to spend any time in the emergency department, as by the time I got to the hospital, my regular room on the CF ward had opened up. Both the doctors and I knew I was going to be in for a long hospital stay, but the hope was that throughout the long stay, I could get more and more healthy and that the month or more of being hospitalized would help beat back the infections and get me as healthy as possible for transplant. This was planned to be a big push to extend my life until I could get my transplant.

I was put on a combination of two antibiotics that had worked well in January and that had given me the month at home during the Olympics. The first week of treatment produced good results, and by the beginning of the second week, I was still on track. Then things stalled, and all progress stopped. The effectiveness of the medications seemed to have worn off; the enemy had outflanked the antibiotics and built new defenses.

Seeing this, my doctors decided to change course and throw something different at the menacing enemy by starting me on a new drug. However, over the next week, we continued to lose ground as things went from bad to worse. Once again, my doctors tried to tilt the battle ground to our favor, this time by giving me a week-long pulse of steroids to try to bring down the growing inflammation in my lungs and therefore have easier access to the bacteria that had now fortified itself deep in my airways. A week later, we found ourselves regrouping again as this course of action was also not having the desired effect.

I had now been in hospital for four weeks, a week longer than any previous admission, and we were no closer to getting me healthier than the day I was admitted. By April 1, I was back on one of the original antibiotics they took me off, as the second one was discontinued, and they were trying another one I had never had in intravenous form before. That day I wrote: *I am quite anxious and frustrated by how things are going. This is totally new ground for us. Usually I come in and they start my meds, and three weeks later, I am feeling better, but this time it has become much more complicated.*

A week later, on April 7, there were some small signs of progress but not much. The doctors did not want to change things up again for fear of exposing me to too many antibiotics, so instead we decided to increase the dose of both drugs I was on. Then the shit hit the fan!

April 8, 2010: *I have not slept much at all the past two nights. My heart rate has been quite high over the past couple days, so they are going to look into that today. I also began breaking out in very itchy hives whenever I was getting my antibiotics. I am getting Benadryl now, but it doesn't seem to be doing too much. I think some more decisions will need to be made tomorrow. For now, it is very annoying.*

Unfortunately, we didn't have a chance to discuss any changes the following day. What happened on April 9, 2010, was one of the scariest moments during my transplant wait. I woke up from snoozing all night to feeling incredibly out of breath. My heart rate was racing. Due to some coincidence on the ward, my nurse did not come in right away after shift change to see how I was doing, so I spent the first 60 to 90 minutes of the day alone in my room.

I went to the bathroom and found that taking the four steps to the toilet was almost impossible. On my way to sitting on the far side of my bed, instead of walking around it, I just flopped onto it and rolled over. I was too out of breath to walk the five steps to the other side.

I knew something was off, but in my brain fog I didn't call my nurse. I figured I just needed to do some physio to clear what I thought was a lot of mucus in my airways. But as I began doing my physio, I found myself hardly even able to do it. After any cough, it took me minutes to catch my breath. At this point, I knew something was *very* wrong. Around 8:15 a.m., my physiotherapist came to my room to check on me and if I needed help with my physiotherapy. By this point, she knew me very well, as each week we were spending a good four to six hours together. I remember turning as my hospital room door opened, seeing her and the look on her face once she fully focused on me. Without saying hi or exchanging any pleasantries, as we always do, she inquired how I was feeling. I shook my head and whispered, "I think something's wrong." With that, she turned on her heel, ran to the nearest hallway phone and called the on-call CF doctor, telling him to get to my room as soon as possible. She then rushed back in and knelt down beside me, trying to figure out what was happening.

She was listening to my breathing and trying to coax out of me what I was exactly feeling. But I was so out of breath that I was finding it near impossible to even talk. It was taking all my energy to suck enough oxygen into my lungs that I was too out of breath to speak.

The CF doctor came rushing into my room within minutes. He took a quick listen to my lungs, gathered the relevant information from my physiotherapist, and, knowing that my medication doses had been upped in the last two days, rushed out to the nursing station. He loaded up a syringe of hydrocortisone, a steroid hormone used to treat inflammation, and injected it into a small bag of fluid hooked up to my IV, then told my nurse to run it in as fast as possible. He also ordered an X-ray, stat!

Before the porter appeared to take me down for the X-ray, my doctor explained that if they couldn't reverse the allergic reaction, I was most likely going to need to be intubated. I *should* start feeling the effects of the steroids within the half hour, but if not, they would need to take very aggressive action.

It was at this moment that I became terrified. I felt that if I could consciously fight, I could get through this and get things back on track, but if I was intubated, I knew that this could spell the beginning of a very quick end for me, because once intubated, your status on the transplant list is suspended. (Note: This was the case in 2010, but is not the case today.)

I was taken down to get an X-ray and made to stand as best I could in front of the X-ray machine while still unable to catch my breath. It had now been about 15 minutes since they started running the steroids into me. I was put back in my wheelchair and wheeled into the hallway, where the porter would pick me up. As I sat there waiting, I started to feel a relaxing in my lungs. It was as if someone was loosening a belt that had been winched around my chest. It was one of the most freeing moments I had felt, similar to when the chest tubes were put in and my lung reinflated. My lungs began relaxing, and air seemed to flow in and out of them again. I was brought back up to my room, and I felt that any talk of intubation wouldn't need to go any further, at least at this point.

The two antibiotics I was on were both stopped immediately, and I was put on another drug, a single antibiotic that was very safe, but which they had been hoping to leave as a last resort for me. They also kept up the hydrocortisone treatment for the rest of the day whenever the effect of the allergic reaction would reappear.

Five days later, after everything had calmed down and my body was given a couple of days of rest from any heavy drugs, my doctors decided to challenge one of the drugs I was on when I had the reaction. I had always done well on this drug, and the doctors wanted to know if they could continue to use it. We started very slowly, and it went fine. Ten days after the reaction and five days into the new drug cocktail I was now on, I started hitting on all cylinders again.

April 19, 2010: *Never did I think I would feel this good again, especially this fast. In no way am I out of the woods, but comparing this last weekend to the previous one is like black and white. I was able to go to the gym on both Saturday and Sunday, which I have not done in over three weeks, and I was able to go on the treadmill again, very slow of course, but it felt so good to be able to walk for 15 minutes. The gym also just got a new rowing machine so I was able to spend five minutes on that as well, and boy, did that feel good on my shoulders! Saturday afternoon, we were able to get out on a pass, so we went home for a couple hours and relaxed watching a movie. On the way back to the hospital, we drove through Stanley Park and took some pictures at Prospect Point. It was a beautiful evening.*

A week later, April 26, Kim and I celebrated our second wedding anniversary. I was let out on a pass for the evening. We drove to Granville Island and splurged on a fancy and expensive dinner. The food was amazing, but at that point, any restaurant food would have been amazing, as I had been eating hospital food the previous seven weeks. I was way underdressed in jeans and a shirt that no longer fit me because of all the weight I had lost, and of course, I also had my mini O2 tank with me. Over dinner, we reflected on how much had happened in our first two years of marriage and how far things had gone off track from what we expected. On the day of our marriage, we knew that a transplant would be in my future, but we never imagined it would happen this soon and that we would have spent so many nights apart this early in our marriage. However, despite the life we were now living, we were both thankful that we were together, walking this journey side-by-side, and despite the situation, we did indeed celebrate the two years we had had together.

That same day, my doctors surprisingly started talking about the possibility of sending me home. We knew that going home was more about taking a break from the drugs and hospital environment than it was about the state of my lungs, but Kim and I were feeling that even if I slipped a bit, it would still be worth it to get out of the hospital for a couple of days.

That day also marked seventeen months that I had been waiting for transplant, but at this point, I found it better to not keep count. I noted the anniversary in my mind, but other than that, let it pass unnoticed.

It was finally on May 5 that I was given the green light to go home. It had been twenty-five days since the allergic reaction that almost put me on a respirator, and it was twenty-one days since the right drug cocktail had finally been found. My doctors and I knew I was going to be back in hospital soon enough, but it was important to allow my body to have breaks when it could afford it.

In total, that admission lasted nine weeks. I am not going to mention the names of the drugs I was all on, as armchair critics and more recent research may critique some of the decisions made, but this is how my medication schedule looked over those nine weeks:

Mar. 5: Admitted to St. Paul's: Started Drug 1 and Drug 2.
Mar. 23: Switch Drug 1 for Drug 3.
Mar. 29: Taken off Drug 3 and put back on Drug 1
at higher frequently.
April. 1: Taken off Drug 2 put on Drug 4.
April 6: Drug 4 dose increased.

April 8: Allergic reaction begins to Drug 4.

April 9: Heavy inflammation in lungs, and all drugs immediately stopped; given a high dose of steroids to bring down inflammation. Consideration is given to be intubated on a respirator.

April 9: Drug 5 started by itself.

April 13: Challenge the allergy: put back on Drug 1 while continuing Drug 5.

The Last Admission

May 17, 2010: (Twelve days after coming home) *There are usually two reasons why a sick person doesn't post on their blog for a long time. They are either feeling really good and enjoying life too much to want to sit and blog, or they are sick and just don't want to talk about it. Well, for me, it started out as the first and then flip-flopped to the second. I will be heading back into St. Paul's today. Same old thing, not much new to say.*

The clinic called and said they had a room ready for me in the early afternoon. As Kim packed my bags, little did we know this would be the last time we would do this. The next time I would see our home, I would be breathing with new lungs!

I should clarify something about the word *home*. Although I just used it to refer to our house, by this point in 2010, I had actually come to see St. Paul's as my home. So far that calendar year, I had spent three weeks in hospital in January, four weeks at home in February, nine weeks in from March to early May, twelve days at home in the middle of May, and now I was going back in. St. Paul's Hospital was no longer my home-away-from-home, but

The Narrowing of Life

it had become my *home*. I was now more comfortable living in hospital than I was living in our house.

While in hospital, I was doing over six hours of physio a day. Twice a day, morning and afternoon, my physiotherapist would come and perform percussion physio on me (remember that, from my childhood). In the evening, Kim would often take this job on herself before leaving for the night. I would lie in different positions on my bed and coach Kim in trying to beat the stubborn mucus out of my lungs. This was the only way I would have any chance of falling sleep. On the days when Kim needed a night off, the on-call physio would come in and do the percussions on me.

By this time, my skin had turned gray due to lack of oxygen in my blood. I could no longer concentrate enough to read. I could not walk, shower, sit, or lie down without supplemental oxygen. I could not sleep for more than 45 minutes at a time before the mucus would plug my upper airways, and I would wake up in a coughing fit. I was also suffering from permanent hearing damage in my right ear because of the side effects of one of the antibiotics I was on (a constant ringing, or tinnitus, which I still have today). And all the while, my transplant was not coming.

One metaphor I kept using when people asked me how I was feeling is that I felt like I was on a sinking ship and the rescue boat from the shore had been dispatched, but I had no clue if it was going to make it on time. All the while, the deep, dark water kept getting closer and closer as the ship was becoming more and more submerged, listing more and more quickly past the point of no return.

The first two-and-a-half weeks of this admission were a slow go. I had slipped back quite a bit in my twelve days at home. We stayed on the same antibiotic cocktail that had finally turned things around during my previous admission, and though there were signs it was working, it was taking its sweet time.

Big Breath In

My physio checked in on me during my second day in hospital, did a quick assessment, and told me she would check in again in a week—it would take at least that long to get me back to a place where I could work out in the gym. She came faithfully to do percussion physio, but there was no talk of the gym for almost two weeks. Finally, in early June, I was back on the treadmill, oxygen blowing through my nasal prongs, almost turned up to the max.

It was also at this time that the lead CF doctor called a family meeting. On a Friday morning in early June, around 11:00 a.m., myself, Kim, my parents, and my sister and brother-in-law, plus the whole CF clinical team, gathered in one of the conference rooms of the hospital.

It is usually never a good sign when a family meeting is called, as issues of mortality usually need to be talked about. It was time to fill in or renew my DNR form, and express my wishes for what kind of heroics I wanted performed if things took a sudden turn for the worse. I don't remember the answers we gave for each question, but basically, the gist was that as long as transplant was on the table, I'd want everything possible done. If I found myself taken off the transplant list for whatever reason and the infections in my lungs sent me into the sudden spiral that was irreversible, then I'd move to comfort care.

The doctor then updated us on my condition. What this update boiled down to was that it was getting critically important that I get my transplant soon. He showed us some charts and graphs of my health, and said we were entering a stage of the illness, an end stage, where everything could unravel in a very short period of time.

It was at this point that I saw my chance to press my doctor for an answer to a question I had begun asking him every once in a while, but which he always evaded answering. *In his medical opinion, based on his experience and what he saw in me, how long did I have to live*? I tried to make it as clear as possible that I was not going to hold it against him if he was wrong, but I wanted, *I needed*, a ballpark time frame on what I had left. For me, information is power, and I have always wanted to know the most I could about what I was facing, even if the news was not good. My doctor once again tried to dodge the question with doctor-speak about how every patient is different, which is very true. I came back at him again, though, this time emphasizing his experience and what he saw in me. He tried evading once again, but I pressed once more. By this time, and having now spent so much time in hospital, I knew my doctors all respected me. I knew they were all rooting for me, and I knew they did not solely see me as a patient but as a real person with inherent dignity, someone who loves and is loved, someone with hopes and dreams but who also accepts the reality he is facing. The truth was, no one, not my CF doctors or even my transplant doctors, had expected me to have to wait this long. There were people who had waited longer than I had, but they also thought it would have already happened for me. Therefore, in seeing I wasn't going to back down from my question, my doctor looked me in the eyes and answered straight. "In four months, you will most likely be too sick for transplant, and I don't think you will have more than two months after that."

That was it. Plain and simple. Rip the bandage off, let it sting, and then move on. And that was what we did. I now knew what I was up against. I now knew how to better pace myself, and I was actually able to calm down. Four months. I had to work my ass off for four months in the hopes my transplant would come in that time. At this point, it was clear that without a transplant I would not live long enough to see the changing of another calendar.

A week after that family meeting, I was getting my legs under me again. The antibiotic cocktail I was on seemed to be getting the upper hand on the bacteria that was fortified in my airways. I was back in the CF gym five times a week, walking on the treadmill for a good fifteen minutes. Kim and I were getting out on the weekends for afternoon passes, but we were staying in Vancouver. We didn't go to our house anymore—that was too far to go for my medication schedule—but we enjoyed some of the drivable sights of the city.

It was also at this time, in mid-June, that I found myself one day walking into the CF gym and commenting to my physio, "If I could just get my transplant *now*, I feel I am in such a good place." After the long uptake of antibiotics and the four weeks I had been in hospital, I was actually feeling quite well. *If I can get my transplant right now, before things take an inevitable turn for the worse, it will be such good timing.* But the days continued to tick by.

June 17, 2010

I have often wondered what it would be like if I had a watch that counted down to the day of my death. What would I feel? What would I say to those I love? How would I prepare myself? Not long ago, a friend of mine led me through a life-reflection exercise. He took out a bag of beads and told me to pick one whose color combination best represented my life. He then asked me to explain why I chose the bead I did. After this, he took out a string, threaded the bead onto the string, and tied a knot at each end. Holding the string by each end, with the bead bobbing in the middle, he talked about how if this string represented the days of our life, we never know where we are on the string. As I sit here today, writing this book at the age of thirty-nine, maybe the bead is in the middle of the string, and I have another thirty-nine years to go. More realistically, as someone with CF who has had a double-lung transplant, that bead is much farther along the string than the halfway point.

The Narrowing of Life

If tragedy should strike, the bead could almost be at the very end of the string without my knowing it. The reality is, we never know where we are at in terms of our journey, so we have to decide, then, how we will live in this unknown future.

Though I never used this kind of language or metaphor while waiting for my transplant, I would frequently wonder where I was in terms of my wait for transplant. Was the bead getting anywhere near the end of the string? Was I halfway through waiting? Did the end of the string even have a knot on it, or would the bead plummet to the ground one day as my lungs filled with fluid.

Though I knew full well that the wait could take up to two years, in the early days, I never imagined I would see the six-month mark; surely it would come before that! So, with that said, as I passed the eighteen-month mark in May 2010 and the wait kept going into its nineteenth month, I wondered, especially after the family visit, would I see the two-year anniversary of being wait-listed? My two-year anniversary would coincide almost perfectly with the six months my doctors said I had left.

Therefore, on June 17, when Kim decided she needed an evening off from coming into the hospital, I agreed that this was a good thing, as it would give me some time to reflect and motivate myself once again for the fight ahead. To do this, I thought I would try to motivate myself by watching the movie *Invictus*, a story of the South African rugby team who were given very little chance in the 1995 World Cup. The movie carries with it the themes of racism, reconciliation, and peace, but for me at the time, it exuded an ethos of inspiration and hope—that maybe what seems impossible in the moment is in fact possible, and that new life could triumph in the face of overwhelmingly negative odds.

As I finished watching the movie, finished up my physio, had my 10:00 p.m. meds hung, brushed my teeth, and hacked up enough mucus to finally allow me to lie down for an hour and get some sleep, a feeling of peace and contentment came over me. Little did I know, however, that as that feeling came over me, and I drifted off to sleep, the bead of my transplant wait finally touched the end of the string.

15.
THE CALL

"Now the hour bows down, it touches me, throbs metallic, lucid and bold: my senses are trembling. I feel my own power—on the plastic day I lay hold."

(*The Book of Hours,* Rainer Maria Rilke)

JUNE 18, 2010, at 5:00 a.m., I awoke from my regular restless sleep to the click of my hospital room door handle and the slow *whoosh* the door sweep made as it opened. The morning dim and fading lights of the downtown Vancouver skyline met my eyes. I often slept with the curtains open as I enjoyed looking at the lights of the surrounding buildings as I fell asleep and awoke again often during the night. A light plodding of sneakers on the floor met my ears as someone walked into the room. Glancing at my wristwatch, I could make out by the light from the hallway that it was 5:00 a.m. I closed my eyes again. This 5:00 a.m. routine had been happening every day for the past four and a half weeks: time for my nurse to hang my first antibiotic for the day.

However, unlike every other morning, when I'd hear the soft shuffle of feet head straight over to the right side of my bed where my IV pole stood, I instead heard the feet coming around the foot of my bed, and a voice saying, "George, are you awake? I need you to wake up."

I opened my eyes again, lifting my head to see my nurse standing at the end of my bed. Then, squinting into the hallway's light, I noticed two other people, both of whom I recognized, one a nurse, the other someone from the IV team. Both were standing in the doorframe with crazy grins on their faces.

I could now see that the nurse standing in front of me had a piece of paper in her hand. By the way she held it and presented it to me, it seemed like it must contain one of the most important or sacred secrets in the world. As she handed me the paper, she blurted out in excitement the four words that I had been yearning to hear for over eighteen months—*eighteen months, three weeks, one day, and fourteen-and-one-half-hours,* to be exact: "Your call has come!" In my 5:00 a.m. daze, I stared back at her, "What?"

"Your call has come . . . the transplant nurse just called," she gushed, with a massive smile on her face. "They found a set of lungs for you. You're going to get your transplant today!"

I looked over to the two people standing in the door, and they were smiling and nodding their heads. I looked back at my nurse, and I could see tears in her eyes. At that moment, as this news sank in—that the potential new life that I had waited so long for was now actually going to happen, and it was going to happen *today*—there was only one emotion I felt: utter gratitude! The finish line had arrived. The rescue boat was drifting alongside. I was going to get my shot!

After those four magical words settled into my being, *"Your call has come,"* the nurse handed me the piece of paper and said to call the number. It was for the pre-transplant coordinator, who was waiting for my call and would give me more information and instructions.

The Call

By this time, reaching for my cell phone, I was in tears, my nurse was in tears, and even the two people at the door were getting teary. I had spent so much time in hospital and on the same ward that all the full-time staff knew my story, knew I was waiting for transplant, and knew that I was getting more and more sick. They were all pulling for me and hoping the transplant would come in time. As I began dialing the number, my nurse left, along with the two people at the door, saying they had to get my chart ready in order to transfer me over to Vancouver General Hospital (VGH), where my transplant would take place.

As I punched the numbers into my phone, slight disappointment passed through my mind that my pager had never actually gone off. I had kind of given up hope that it ever would. I knew that if the call came while I was in hospital, it would go to the nursing station. Still, I had carried this stupid thing around with me for over eighteen months. All it ever did was remain silent and impotent (except for pager testing day every second Thursday). However, the fleeting disappointment was just that: fleeting.

I called the hallowed number on the piece of paper, identified who I was and why I was calling, and the person on the other end said she would transfer me to the lung coordinator.

The line picked up. "Hello, George? We have a set of lungs for you, this is it!" Once again, tears filled my eyes at these sweet life-giving words.

The pre-transplant coordinator filled me in on the details: the organ retrieval team was working on the donor, giving us some time to get everything lined up on this side. They were lining up an ambulance to come to St. Paul's to pick me up, and I should begin packing right away, as they would be there within the hour. If everything continued as planned, the surgery should be around mid-morning. She said the rest of the info would be given to me once I got to VGH. She wished me good luck, said we would be in touch in a couple hours, and then hung up. I knew she had a lot more work to do, as did I.

I took a minute to gather myself, to sit on the edge of my bed and let the reality of everything sink in, to remind myself to *remember this moment*. Things would never be the same, both for myself and for the people I was about to call.

I made a mental note of the people I had to call: Kim, Dad and Mom, my sister and brother-in-law, and Kim's parents. I picked up my phone and realized that I was about to drop the biggest bomb on these unsuspecting people, and I was going to be waking all of them up.

Kim was obviously the first call I made. In getting that call at 5:00 a.m., she later relayed to me, her reaction was twofold. First, she thought something must be wrong and the hospital was calling with bad news. But second, in the instant before picking up, she wondered if this was my call. She picked up and said, "Hello," and before even saying "hi" myself, I just blurted out, "I got the call. I'm getting my transplant!"

I told her to come as quick as possible to St. Paul's as she had some work to do in packing up my room. We didn't know when the ambulance was going to come, but I wanted her to be there for that, as I didn't want to make that ride by myself. However, because I had now been in hospital for almost five weeks, I had accumulated lots of stuff in my room, and I wasn't going to be able to pack it all up myself.

I called my parents next. My mom answered, already awake and getting ready to go to the barn. (My dad was outside working.) When I gave her the news, her reaction was tempered and calm. Obviously, she was very excited, but we knew by this point to not let our highs get too high. Interestingly enough, when the phone rang, my mom thought right away that this could be it. She mentioned that as she was getting ready for work that morning, she was wondering if the transplant would happen that coming weekend. (It was a Friday morning.) This was not a thought that she'd had any other Friday morning, but for some reason, her spirit was burning, wondering if this might, in fact, be the weekend it would happen.

I then called my sister, Lynette. She had just finished her shift in the ICU at VGH the day before. As we talked, I could hear a mixture of relief and excitement in her voice, but also a weighed tone of anxiety filtered through the receiver. She said that she and Bryan would meet me at the hospital in a couple of hours, once I had been transferred and things had settled down a bit. Having worked in the intensive care unit for almost a decade, Lynette had seen the best of what a transplant could do, but she had also seen the worst.

I knew and sensed throughout the whole waiting period that Lynette carried a special and very heavy burden for me. She was born into a vocation of caring for others. From a very young age, she instinctively became a caregiver for Warren as she witnessed his hardship and sickness. With my parents caring for two chronically ill sons, Lynette was shaped and formed into someone who often needed to find her own inner strength to rise above the difficulty and hardship she saw around her. Instead of stomping her feet and demanding more attention for herself, she instead jumped right in as a protector and caregiver for both myself and Warren.

With my mom having trained as a nurse and often telling us nursing stories in our younger years, and with Lynette's natural aptitude and formation as a caregiver, it was a natural step for her to go to nursing school straight out of high school. Lynette's place to shine was always at the bedside, seeking the most acute areas and patients that her training would allow. Upon graduation from nursing school, she got a job at VGH, on the floor where she did her practicum and where I would eventually find myself after transplant, the thoracic ward. After a number of years there, cutting her bedside teeth with patients recovering from surgery or other respiratory ailments, she would apply for critical care training and get a job in the intensive care unit, where she excelled once again in her work, often being in charge of the most critically ill patients in the unit, if not the whole province.

When it came to my transplant, it was through some of the most formative and self-identifying parts of herself that she experienced it: loving and concerned sister, and critical care nurse. Her place of work was where I would end up immediately after surgery; it would be the place where my new life would begin; but it could also be, like she had seen times before with her patients, the place where I could languish for weeks, if not months, not being able to get off the ventilator, my body wasting away and wracked with infection, or the ultimate danger of acute and sudden rejection. While I was in the ICU and with my transplant now in progress, it meant that Lynette would not be able to return to work until after I was out of the ICU. Having me in there as a critically ill patient would create too much of a distraction and potential conflict of interest for her, so she would have to take time off. Therefore, this phone call I was making, letting her know my transplant was on, signaled the end of work for her until I had recovered enough to get out of her workplace, whenever that might be. As I talked with Lynette on the phone that early morning, I was not the only one with incredible unknowns in front of me. My phone call placed her in a very precarious situation with a wide spectrum of anxiety and joy flowing through her.

Lastly, I called Kim's parents. As the phone was ringing, I suddenly realized that this was only the second time I was calling their house to just talk to them. The only other time I had done this was when

I called to ask them out for coffee, wanting to seek their blessing as I intended to ask Kim to marry me. They were so excited to receive my call (about the transplant ☺).

During this time, my nurse came in and out of my room, asking questions, doing sets of vitals, giving me my physio meds, and trying to get everything confirmed with the paramedics and VGH. (You can see why I didn't get much packing done myself.)

Kim arrived at 5:45, and at the same time, my nurse let us know it would still be a while before the ambulance could come to pick me up. Because this was not an emergency, I would have to wait until one became available.

With some of the time pressure now off, Kim began packing up the room in a bit more of a relaxed state. Usually, when I got discharged, Kim would start packing and taking stuff home a day or two in advance, so it was not such a big load on the day I was released. Of course, now it all had to go in one shot, and she ended up having to make three trips down to the car to empty the whole room. It pretty much filled her whole trunk and some of the back seat. But as she finished and came back upstairs, it now being about 6:30 a.m., we sat on the edge of the bed and once again waited. I told her about the phone calls I'd made and everyone's reaction, and she told me about her first thoughts when her phone rang. Finally, at 7:00 a.m., two paramedics appeared at my door with a stretcher in tow.

Hospital Transfer

The wait for the ambulance should have been the first sign that the romanticized speed and drama that I was told would accompany transplant-day were not going to be part of my experience. I have

Big Breath In

talked to others for whom this had been part and parcel of their great life-changing day, but this would not be my story. Mine can be much better described as a patience-building exercise.

When the paramedics showed up, I saw right away that this was going to be a very slow show, as along with the two guys at my door, was a third—the dreaded trainee! Now don't get me wrong, I have nothing against training people and on-the-job mentoring; it is part of the medical field training, and it is a good thing. However, when someone has been waiting for over a year and a half for the chance of a life-saving transplant with untold possibilities, every second of delay after the green light has been given is like torture!

The captain of the three-man crew first took the trainee over to the nursing station to begin the paperwork, and in doing so, saw this as the perfect opportunity to do some teaching. At this point, I was hunched over, standing in the hallway with Kim and the second paramedic. We stood in the hallway for a good ten minutes as the paperwork was sorted out. The trainee got a good education in medical charts and the pages they would need to transfer me to the other hospital. As we stood there, staring longingly at the nursing station, trying to will the captain and trainee to get this show on the road, the much more causal paramedic standing with us kept apologizing for the delay, loudly asking down the hallway, "What's the hold up over there?" Both Kim and I liked him.

After about fifteen minutes of standing around waiting, we finally started heading for the elevators. I was repeatedly asked if I wanted to go down in a wheelchair or stretcher, but my pride asserted itself. As a testament to everything I had gone through in the previous year and a half, and as a show of appreciation for all the amazing work the nurses did in keeping me going, I was determined to walk out of that hospital on my own two feet. (Of course, with the help of an oxygen tank.)

The Call

We made our way outside, and I was put in the bucket seat in the back of the ambulance. Kim also got to ride in the back with me. At this point with my health, I was much more comfortable sitting up than lying down, as anytime I lay down, it shifted the mucus in my lungs, moving it higher in my airways and causing a coughing attack that would last for minutes.

By car, the distance between St. Paul's Hospital and VGH is only about ten minutes, but I'll be damned if that wasn't the longest ride I have ever taken. I could swear that the ambulance driver took every detour he could think of, as I saw parts of the city I had never seen before (however, I was sitting backward, and everything looks a bit different when sitting that way in an ambulance).

It was a very strange feeling to be at street level among all those cars and people. Other than some weekend afternoon passes, I had not been off the ward for almost five weeks. But as we drove to VGH, I couldn't help but think of how strange and surreal all this was. Here were people going to work in their BMWs, Honda Civics, and Range Rovers, all trying to beat the traffic, grabbing some breakfast and a coffee before hitting the office, and right beside them in traffic was me, sitting in the back of an ambulance on what was the most transformative day of my life.

It was as if I was holding a massive secret. As I passed within feet of these people, everyone in professional office attire, or construction workwear, here I was, sitting in my PJs, hooked up to oxygen, entering a twenty-four-hour period where the trajectory of my life was going to completely change. Within hours, my lungs were going to be removed from my body and replaced with another person's lungs, and the world was going on as if nothing out of the ordinary was happening.

Big Breath In

When we arrived at VGH, I finally agreed to get on the stretcher. The paramedics told me it was going to be a long walk to get to where we needed to go and the admitting process might take a while. As they opened the back door of the ambulance, I was hit with the smell of the exhaust fumes from the covered Emergency Department drop-off area and it sent me into a short coughing fit. These lungs of mine were finished.

We came in through the ER doors, and it was clear they were expecting us. We were ushered straight through the waiting area and told to head upstairs right away. It was quite the journey through many back hallways and restricted doors to finally get to the elevators. Then the obligatory wait for an elevator, and of course, we ended up hitting almost every floor as we ascended.

Arriving on the twelfth floor, I was wheeled into a room with an amazing view of south Vancouver. Again, as I looked out the window, all I could think about was that in those hundreds of houses out there, people were starting their day like any other. But for me, today signaled my chance to one day join them again in ordinary life, through the gift of a double-lung transplant.

The paramedics wished me all the best in what lay ahead as they helped me off the stretcher and into the hospital bed. A nurse showed up and began a saline drip to keep me hydrated, as I was not able to eat or drink anything. The nurse said they would begin the anti-rejection regimen within the hour so that my immune system would already be blunted when the new lungs were hooked up.

Excitement was high at this point. I called my parents, and they insisted on coming right away, as did Lynette and Bryan. Kim and I sat with eager anticipation, thinking that we were only an hour or two away from surgery. *Will my family even make it in time to see me?* However, little did we know we were now beginning what would be the longest day of our lives!

16.
THE LONGEST DAY

"Between the idea and the reality
Between the motion and the act
Falls the Shadow"

("The Hollow Men," T.S. Eliot)

DURING MY FIRST two hours at VGH, I got busy doing physio. I also had a lot of blood work done, and I mean *a lot*. The technician came to see me twice and, each time, drew more blood than I had ever had taken in one sitting before.

In the lead-up to surgery, though everything looked good on paper, the doctors had to check, double-check, and triple-check that the donor and recipient were as good a match as possible. There is a lot the doctors can do through medications to give the recipient the best chance possible of accepting the lungs, and looking at blood counts is the best way to know what the recipient needs for this to happen. My parents showed up within an hour of me and Kim arriving at VGH, and Lynette and Bryan soon followed.

Within those first couple of hours after arrival, I talked to the transplant coordinator again. She had been up throughout night consulting with the donor's surgeon, my transplant surgeon, and my transplant medical doctors. My surgeon also came in to see me, chat about any anxiety I was having, and explain the process once more. Surgery would probably be in the early afternoon.

At around 11:30 a.m., we found out that things were not going as fast as first thought and the surgery would be moved back to later afternoon, probably 5:00 (twelve hours after the call had come). With this new bit of information, my parents went home for a couple of hours, as there was no use for everyone to just sit there in my small hospital room, staring at each other.

Throughout the day, I started taking my first immunosuppression medications. With this inaugural dose, I began a practice that I have participated in every twelve-hours since that day, religiously taking my meds, thus keeping my natural immune system dulled to the foreign objects now residing in my body. These drugs were, and are, my lifeline, replacing my old antibiotics, which had pretty much run the course of their usefulness. What these first immunosuppression drugs symbolized was a shift in focus and direction in my life, from the disease that was killing me to the hope of new life. Hope finally came to replace the despair we had been feeling for quite some time. As I enthusiastically received this first dose of immunosuppression medication, my life-sustaining antibiotics finally stopped.

I admit I was very nervous about stopping my antibiotics. Rule 101 of antibiotics is you don't stop your antibiotics and then restart them after missing a couple of doses. This is what leads to antibiotic-resistant bacteria. It is also a well-known fact that 30% of all transplant calls are false alarms. This means that everything looks good on paper, but once the donor is in surgery to have their organs removed, the whole process falls apart as the organs are not actually viable. So, I was nervous about missing my antibiotics, knowing that nothing was certain until the surgeon had removed the lungs from my donor. However, I also figured that it must be a good sign that they stopped my antibiotics because this must mean that the transplant was a certainty.

I was also not able to eat or drink anything throughout the day. With no breakfast, and now no lunch, I was thankful that the anticipation of what was coming was leaving me with little to no appetite. Food was one of the furthest things from my mind.

At around 3:30 p.m., my parents came back to the hospital. We knew things could start happening any time now. The organ retrieval was supposed to start at 4:00 p.m., so as the clock struck the top of the hour, the waiting became almost unbearable. At this point, we figured the lungs had been removed and were sitting on ice in a cooler somewhere, deteriorating ever so slightly with each passing minute that blood wasn't flowing through them. Finally, at around 5:00 p.m., my nurse notified me to get ready. It would be any time now.

As you may have picked up by now, my family is not the most emotional or touchy-feely family there is. But I knew this would be a milestone in our collective lives, and I wanted to say something in case things went sideways during surgery. Having changed into my gown and come out of the bathroom, our family read a psalm together from the Bible, Psalm 27. (If you are not familiar with the Bible, a psalm is a poetic prayer.) Psalm 27 is a prayer of trust and peace in God, of waiting for deliverance from struggle.

After reading this, we prayed together that the surgery and recovery ahead would go well and we also said a prayer for my donor and their family. We assumed at this point that my donor, having gone into the organ retrieval surgery, was now fully deceased. They, of course, would have already been declared brain-dead before I got my call at 5:00 a.m. But with the retrieval surgery having taken place, they would have been taken off any life-support measures, and their family would no longer be at the hospital with them. As our family experienced with Warren's passing, leaving your deceased loved one in hospital and driving home to a silent house is a heart-wrenching experience. My parents knew the disarray of these moments and what it is like to know that your loved one is not coming back. Therefore, this moment—in fact, the whole day—was arduous for my parents. Not only were they suffering from the anxiety of what lay ahead for me, but they knew what it was like on the other side of the transplant spectrum, and the death that was involved to give me this new life.

After spending a moment in prayer, remembering the life lived by my donor, I got up and hugged my dad, mom, and Lynette (Bryan had gone home earlier), telling them how much I loved them. It was not something we often did, but I knew I could not go peacefully into my surgery without expressing how much they had all done for me and how much I loved them. We spoke few words after that.

In the silence that followed, our anticipation built. But as we continued to wait, there was also a growing sense of stress and foreboding. Every footstep outside my hospital room, every stretcher that came down the hallway, was a moment of emotional rise and fall, hoping that the approaching sound would stop at my door. But that hope crashed each time the footsteps or stretcher passed by.

Finally, an hour after being told to get ready, Lynette, who knew the floor like the back of her hand, went to try to find out what was happening. What she learned was that there had been an emergency, and the operating room was needed. The transplant had been delayed.

On hearing this news, we tried to be rational and calm. Obviously, a true emergency was happening, and someone would die if they were not operated on right away. This *was* more urgent than my transplant, but our anxiety only grew, as we were under the impression that the lungs I was going to receive were just sitting on ice somewhere.

The minutes, and then hours slowly kept passing. Kim and I would lock eyes every couple of minutes, a faint smile would pass between us, but we didn't venture too much more hope than that. We were trying to hold the delicate balance of preparing for the worst, but still holding onto the best. At around 7:30 p.m., with nothing happening, Lynette decided to go home as there was nothing else to do and it had been a long day already. I admit I was surprised by her leaving, but I also knew that Bryan had been home since the late morning, anxiously awaiting any news.

Bryan is an amazing brother-in-law. He carries so many of our family burdens, and I knew that being ninety minutes away and having to work (he is also a farmer) was not easy for him that day. It was good Lynette went home to be with him, but I was also wondering if this tension and waiting were getting to her. She had a wealth of experience with lung transplants and she knew how these things could go and how they could go wrong. I wondered if she could see the red flags appearing throughout the day, and that in her own fragility, she knew she couldn't be at the hospital if the bad news of a cancelled surgery had to be delivered.

It was now 8:00 p.m., fifteen hours since getting the call and four hours since we thought the lungs had been retrieved. We were still optimistic I would be going in soon, but our world was about to fall apart.

At around 8:15, my transplant surgeon knocked on the door frame of my hospital room and came in for what we expected to be our final briefing before surgery. But as he walked up to my bedside, it was not a look of anticipation on his face, but one of sorrow and concern. A down-to-earth man, he spoke straight but also with a deep sense of compassion. He informed us that the transplant was most likely not going to happen. He said my donor lungs had not yet been retrieved because just before they were about to retrieve them, they began failing. The donor surgeon had been working very hard on saving them since 4:00 p.m., but they were continuing to fail. It was likely that my transplant would not be happening. This was going to be a dry run. He said that the retrieving surgeon was incredibly talented and still had a couple of things to try, but the lungs had gone from functioning around 95% down to 30%. In this state, they were no longer suitable for transplant.

Kim and I were able to hold it together while our surgeon was in the room. We thanked him for coming up to inform us in person, but as soon as he left, I collapsed on the bed and wept. Somehow, I knew this was my shot. This was my one shot and I had just lost it. We had come so close, waited so long, had gone through so much, and all the while my health kept slipping away. I had been waiting fifteen hours since my call, and now it had slipped through our fingers. It was at this point, a little after 8:00 p.m., on June 18, 2010, that I finally gave up. I lost all hope. As I lay on the bed, trying to take deep breaths between sobs, I tried as hard as I could to picture going back to St. Paul's, of starting the wait all over again, slipping back in my routine, facing all the nurses and doctors and their sympathetic looks. I knew I wouldn't be able to do it. To come so close at this late stage in my health, and now to have to go back onto all the antibiotics and physio, knowing that without transplant, the best-case scenario was that I had about three-and-half months left before I would be too sick for surgery, anyway. What was the point of trying any longer? I didn't have it in me anymore.

My parents had gone for a quick dinner before my surgeon had visited us with this news. When they came back, we told them

The Longest Day

what had happened. We all sat for about thirty minutes in total silence, all thinking the same thing: we had just lost our shot.

I phoned my sister and let her know; it seemed her premonition had been right. It was best she wasn't there. My dad stepped out of the room to call my uncle and my grandma, to try to explain to them what had gone so wrong.

After about an hour, which my dad would later call "the worst hour of our lives," I was able to collect my thoughts enough to decide that if this transplant wasn't happening, then I wanted something to eat and I wanted to go home. I knew that St. Paul's wasn't holding my room. Besides, I had been feeling better over the past week, and so I wanted to go home. If this was the end of the road, if I had really missed my chance, then I wanted one more extended time in our house, away from medications and all the rest. I was going to let my health drop as low as I could stand it and then admit myself to St. Paul's for what I knew would be the last time.

I rang my call bell and asked my nurse to tell my doctors that I would like something to eat and drink. He said he would give my surgeon a call to see where things stood. Once we got the final word then we could get things going in terms of food, drink, and going home. About five minutes later, the nurse came back and said my surgeon was on the phone in the hallway and he was asking for a member of the family. I nodded at my mom to take the call, as in this vulnerable state, I couldn't stand not having Kim at my side, even for a moment. About a minute later, my mom came back in the room, with tears in her eyes and a look of anticipation. "The transplant is back on," she said. "It's a go!"

In a last-ditch effort to save the lungs, the recovery surgeon opened up the chest cavity of my donor and began manually working on the lungs, suctioning the accumulating fluid in and around the lungs. I don't know all the details, but by opening up the chest cavity and manually working on the lungs, the recovery surgeon was able to get them working back up to 75%, within reason for transplant.

However, the final choice to receive the lungs in this condition was mine. The lungs were no longer perfect; in fact, they were now permanently damaged. My surgeon came back to the floor, informed us of the circumstance, and asked if we wanted to proceed. I could tell by his own voice and body language that he thought it was safe to go ahead. In reality, based on what we experienced in the previous hour, I needed no convincing. When the question came, I didn't even think about it, but instead jumped in with an emphatic *YES!*

Within five minutes of this news and consenting to go ahead with the surgery, there was a stretcher outside my door, ready to take me down to the pre-op room. Wearing nothing but a very thin hospital gown, under any other circumstance, I would have been quite sheepish, cold, and a little self-conscious being wheeled down those halls. But at this point, my adrenaline was pumping so hard that I could have been stark-naked in the middle of a snowstorm, surrounded by 20,000 people, and I still could not have cared less.

Not being familiar with the hospital, it seemed like a neverending journey through hallway after hallway, with Kim and my parents following close behind. Finally, we came through a set of double doors and into the pre-operating room. It was a very large, open square room. On the ground were markings like a parking lot, showing where each bed, during the busy hours, should be parked as people waited for their surgeries. Because it was late on a Friday night and there are no surgeries scheduled for that time, the room stood deserted and dark, except for one parking spot in the far corner, beside two big doors that said, "Operating

Rooms: Authorized Persons Only." Under any other circumstance, this would have been a spooky and eerie room to stumble into late at night, but we only had one thing on our minds, and that was getting into that OR!

As the porter stationed my bed in parking stall one, another set of doors to my left opened. A woman came in and introduced herself as the anesthesiologist. She had my file with her. We went over a couple of questions having to do with allergies and a couple of things that would be happening while I was still awake in the operating room. Then, of course, there were the forms to sign, consenting in writing to what I had consented to verbally upstairs. My signature is illegible at the best of times, so I can only imagine at this point what squiggly line I scrolled across the page. She left, and within a minute, another person came in, asking similar questions and said I would be going in a couple of minutes.

I asked Kim to take two quick pictures: one of me alone, and then one of me and my parents. I said my goodbyes to my dad and mom. After that, they took a couple of steps back, and I said my goodbyes to Kim. Neither Kim or I had much understanding of what we were getting into when we had married just two years earlier, of the shifts that life would bring within our first years together, but Kim had stuck by my side the entire time. After we said our goodbye and shared a last kiss, two porters appeared through the door and said they were ready to take me in. They wheeled me around to face the large "Authorized Persons Only" doors. I waved back at Kim and simply said, "See you in a bit." The porters wheeled me through the doors, took a sharp turn to the left, and picked up speed down the long hallways. It was on!

Operating Room

As the doors closed behind us, leaving Kim and my parents behind to wait out the night in anxious anticipation, the porters pushed my stretcher down the hallway at a light jog—this was serious! As we passed door after door leading to different operating rooms and who knows what else, I saw a set of open doors on the right, at the end of the hallway. Light streaming out of them. *That must be it,* I thought.

As we approached the open doors, the porters slowed to a walk. We rounded the corner, and I got my first look at the room where the most pivotal moment of my life would occur, and for which I would be unconscious the whole time.

For some reason, in all my daydreaming of what this day might be like, I had never pictured the operating room, but here I was, the place where miracles happen. And what was awaiting me was like something out of a movie set. A bright, clean room, spacious if not for the multitude of machines, trays, tubes, and people that over the next eight hours would have one goal: keeping me alive and ushering me into the next chapter of my life.

My bed came to a stop beside what looked like an overly large metal tray. The fact that it was in the center of the room with a very large bright light hanging over it brought me to the conclusion that this would be my bed for the coming night. I was helped onto the surgical table and laid down on my back, my oxygen tubing transferred from the O2 bottle on the stretcher to the OR system. New IVs were hung, and the stretcher I was brought in on was wheeled away. The large OR doors closed like a vault.

Within a minute, I was asked to sit up, swing my legs over the right side of the table, and hunch over so I could have my epidural inserted. I was told to hunch over so the technician—technician is such a cold word, but when someone is inserting a long needle

The Longest Day

into your spine, I find it comforting that their title is technician—could get a good look at my spine. I placed my elbows on my knees, rounded my shoulders, hung my head forward, and prayed that I wouldn't have a coughing fit. However, I need not have worried, for as I hunched over, two strong yet comforting hands held my shoulders tight so that I remained perfectly still. I always find the most painful part of any major medical procedure is the freezing—it stings. This was what I was thinking just minutes before my surgery. A surgery in which my sternum would be separated, my ribs retracted, my chest popped open like the hood of a car. Where my surgeon would cut my lungs out of my body. My chest cavity scraped clean of scar tissue from years of chronic lung infection and two collapsed lungs. Two new lungs would then be placed inside of it. Finally with wire, small rods and stitches, my chest would be sewn back together. "But please, take it easy on the freezing, it stings!"

I didn't feel much of the epidermal going in; there was too much adrenaline pumping and too many thoughts going through my mind. The thing I remember from this moment is the two nursing hands that held my shoulders as it was going in. Something about the human touch in that most-vulnerable moment was so comforting.

Within a couple minutes, the epidural was in and I was once again lying down on my little metal table. The assisting surgeon came over to make sure I was feeling good and didn't have any last-minute questions—not that it would have mattered at this point.

The pace in the OR began picking up, as the surgeons were now in the room, and I was on the table and ready to go to sleep. I wondered what would happen first. I knew I needed to have a lot of IVs inserted. I knew at some point I would need a catheter—please let me be asleep for that insertion! I had no clue what order things would be put in me (or taken out of me) or how I would be prepared for surgery. My wonderings, however, were soon answered as within seconds of the surgeon leaving my side, the anesthesiologist walked into view with a mask in her hand. She asked if she could place it over my nose and mouth and then told me to breathe. As she placed the mask on my face, the smell of rubber hit my nose, with a metallic note of whatever it was that was flowing through the line.

In my final moments of consciousness, I told myself one last time that this was the right thing to do. Without this transplant, I knew I had only months left to live. I told myself that these were the last breaths I would take with the lungs that I was born with. Lungs that came to life and filled with oxygen the moment I was born. Lungs that powered me to take my first steps and that had carried me through elementary school. They allowed me to play ice hockey and run track. Lungs that brought me through high school and gave me the words to flirt with girls and negotiate buying my first car. Through their inflating and deflating, they gave me the strength to work on our family dairy farm and get a bachelor of arts degree. Lungs that allowed me to meet, date, and marry Kim. But they were also lungs that were ticking time bombs. They were filled with scaring and mucus that would soon drown me. Lungs that were pock-marked from chronic infections and that resembled two large stones rather than pink squishy orbs. Lungs that were now killing me. It was time to say goodbye.

They had done their job for twenty-eight years, but the cystic fibrosis that was part and parcel of their DNA had now ravaged them beyond repair. As the anesthetic pulled me across the threshold of consciousness, I prayed one last prayer, thankful for the opportunity to receive this second chance at life.

17.
RECOVERY: DAY 1

"So, here we go in faith. Last words of advice—try to be one with the ventilator!?!? It's going to be hard George, but try to keep the anxiety down & take nice slow breaths—
you'll do great!
And for crying out loud don't pull anything out!
We'll just have to put it back in!

("To be Opened When Pager Goes Off," A letter from Lynette)

JUNE 19, 2010: *Hi, Everyone. This is Kim. After a very long 24 hours, I am very happy to blog for George that he has just had his transplant and is now in the ICU. He is not out of the woods by any means, but the surgery is over and it has finally happened. Thank you for all your prayers. I know this is not very informative and will lead to more questions but eventually George will probably blog out the whole process. Bye for now. Kim*

After I was wheeled out of the pre-op doors and down the long hallways to the operating room, Kim and my parents hung around for about thirty minutes, waiting long enough that I would most likely be asleep and nothing was going to be cancelled at the last minute. They left the hospital around 10:00 p.m., under a beautiful summer night sky. Kim remembers being calm on the drive home, which took about thirty minutes. She unpacked the car, still full of my St. Paul's hospital room belongings, which she had packed in haste some seventeen hours earlier. (My parents had brought her car from St. Paul's to VGH.) She started a load of laundry, watched a bit of TV, grabbed something light to eat, and, around 11:30 p.m., turned out the lights and fell asleep. At 2:00 a.m., the phone rang. She sprang upright in bed, grabbed her cell from the nightstand, and smashed it to her ear.

"Hi, Kim? This is George's surgeon. I had said I would give you a call halfway through surgery to let you know how it is going. Things are going well. We are about halfway through. George is doing well." *Click.*

At this point, in what was meant to be a calming measure by my surgeon, Kim's anxiety shot through the roof. She tried to lie down but began feeling a lump form in her throat. She instinctively reached for her phone to call me, as she usually did when feeling anxious about being at home while I was in hospital, but before picking it up, realized I would not be answering on the other end. In fact, my phone was only meters away from her in the living room. She got up and began to pace. She lay down but shot right back up to her feet. At this point, she knew she couldn't be alone, so she called her parents and asked them to come right over.

Things had finally caught up with Kim. It had now been eighteen months, three weeks, and going-on two-days since I was wait-listed for transplant. I had been wait-listed just seven months into our marriage. It was now the 201st night that Kim had spent alone in our house while I was in hospital. On almost all of those except for a handful, Kim had driven more than 100 kilometres a day to visit me. Each workday, she would get up early, pack me some clothes in a bag, and some food in a cooler. She would then drive to work, put in a full day (although her boss would often let her leave an hour early so she could beat rush hour traffic), and be on time to visit me for dinner. She would bring me new clothes and my dinner, sit with me, eat with me, and often watch some TV with me, often when I was less than entertaining or even cordial. She would often stay until 9:00 p.m. and, before leaving, would give me a back or a leg massage due to my increasing restless leg syndrome. Or she would do the final percussion physio of the day for about thirty minutes, trying to beat the mucus out of me before driving the half hour home. She would do laundry and wash out my dishes when she got home and then go to bed, repeating it all the following day.

She never complained, at least not to me. She never considered not doing it, never thought of leaving me for someone else who would come with a lot more potential in their future and a lot fewer burdens in the present. She did it with strength, perseverance, and an amazing spirit of love and grace. It took until the actual night of my surgery, in the middle of my surgery, picturing me at that moment, chest cracked open, one lung outside of my body, to finally break down and need some help herself.

Her parents arrived in about thirty minutes. She sat and talked with them for an hour. Then she and her mom went for an early morning walk on the dyke path behind our house.

At 6:30 a.m., the phone rang again. The surgery was over. All went well. I was in ICU.

Intensive Care Unit

Light then dark, light then dark, light then dark—this is all I remember of going to sleep and waking up, and I don't know if the visionary light and darkness were from going under or waking up, but I suppose I remembered one of them.

My surgery lasted for eight hours, from 10:00 p.m. on June 18 to 6:00 a.m. on June 19. After being transferred to the ICU at around 6:30 a.m., my surgeon called Kim to tell her everything had gone well. Kim right away called my parents and then my sister. Kim and Lynette decided to meet at VGH at 9:00 a.m., as no visitors would be able to see me before then.

The first time I recall waking up, Kim and Lynette were already in my ICU room, standing at the foot of my bed. It was around 9:30 a.m. The nurses had woken me up earlier, but I can't remember that at all. All I remember from the initial waking up was that I was conscious of where I was, I had a horrible taste in my mouth, all I could smell was the plastic or rubber NG tube in my nose, and I was trying to concentrate on what Lynette had always told me about waking up in ICU, that no matter what, *STAY CALM!*

I don't know how many times she had actually told me that when I woke up in the ICU to allow the ventilator to do all the work and try not to fight it. To allow it to breathe for me. The best way to do that was simple: *stay calm.* She would tell me horror stories of people waking up, freaking out, thinking they couldn't breathe, and yanking out their breathing tube, only to find that then they really couldn't breathe, and then it would have to be inserted again, which is absolute hell. So, she had drilled into me for the past year and a half that when I woke up in the ICU, I had to *STAY CALM!* And it worked. It was also one of the last things I thought of before being put under the night before. *Okay, George.*

Recovery: Day 1

The next time you wake up, no matter what happens, even if you somehow wake up with no lungs in your body, STAY CALM!

This proved to be a very valuable liturgy that was engrained in me, as for those first couple hours of consciousness, whenever I began to get anxious, whenever I began feeling I had trouble breathing, I would just remember what Lynette said, *"Stay calm, you are getting everything your body need through the ventilator. Stay calm . . . stay calm . . . stay calm."*

I have no recollection of the next couple hours, but around 11:30 a.m., I woke up and must have been uncomfortable, as I began to move my head from side to side, shifting a little in my bed. I also remember being extremely thirsty because during surgery, and also now in the ICU, my body was being dried out of any extra fluids in order to reduce the amount of fluid that could end up gathering in and around my new lungs.

As the hours passed, I began waking up more and more, trying to shift around in the bed, as I was becoming more uncomfortable. The breathing tube was also becoming annoying as I was being weened and was having to do more breathing on my own. The only thing more difficult than letting the machine breathe for you is trying to breathe in tandem with it. The *stay-calm* mantra was losing its effectiveness.

At some point in the early afternoon, I must have swallowed hard or something, and my NG tube, which went through my nose and down into my stomach, somehow got curled in my esophagus. I started gagging, which made things even worse. Imagine someone sticking their finger down your throat while you are only about 25% conscious and you already have a large breathing tube going down there. The stay-calm mantra was thrown out the window. I began to rock my head back and forth on my pillow, flapping my hands on the mattress in order to get someone's attention, as of course, I couldn't talk because of the breathing tube.

Big Breath In

My sister was there and right away began asking me questions. My nurse also jumped into action, as she could see I was struggling. She came over and, with perfect calm, shone a flashlight into my mouth and could see the NG tube had curled in the back of my throat. She loosened the tape on my nose, which is supposed to keep the tube in place, and began pulling on it ever so slightly. She pulled it roughly an inch-and-a-half, and the gagging immediately stopped. During this whole process, my sister calmly described to me what was happening, that nothing bad was going to happen, and that this was exactly why I had not been allowed food and drink the previous day.

With all the movement I had been making in the bed, plus my swelling anxiety and the movement of the feeding tube, I now found my breathing tube becoming less and less tolerable. As I mentioned before, for the past couple of hours, my nurse, under my doctor's direction, had begun weaning me off the ventilator, thus allowing me to breathe more on my own. I was now breathing in tandem when the ventilator. Even during this whole gagging episode with the feeding tube, my O2 saturation had not dropped much.

With the NG tube back in position, I now wanted the ventilator out. This, at least back in 2010, was considered too early to come off the vent. I had only been out of surgery for about eight hours, but I could feel something within me telling me I could do this. This wasn't a risk for me; it wasn't an experiment. Something inside of me was telling me it was time that I could begin taking my first breaths with my new lungs.

Now, some post-transplant patients I have spoken with talk about taking in their first big gulps of air with their new lungs. They tell it like they woke up from a wonderful nap, waking to the light, opening their eyes, and deeply breathing in the life-giving oxygen around them. Well, I call bullshit on that! Okay, I shouldn't say that. Who am I to judge someone else's experience? But if those experiences are true, then I am one jealous SOB.

For me, I was in an incredible amount of pain. Half the time, I didn't know if I was waking up or falling asleep. My body was dried out, and I was the thirstiest I had ever been in my life. It was very tough! And yet, *something was different.* As miserable as I felt, I also knew there was something different about my body, something I had not felt in over a decade. My body was feeling a new confidence, a confidence that communicated I could all of a sudden do some work, that I would be able to expel energy that could last for more than a couple minutes. Energy that could last for a couple hours! I felt a sense of life coursing through my veins; I don't know if it was just the oxygen-rich blood, the high steroid dose I was on, the four units of blood I'd needed in the OR, or the extra one I had received in the ICU that morning, but I felt for the first time in years that it was time to get down to some real work of recovery. And I instinctively felt I had the lung capacity to do it.

My respirologist, knowing that everything had gone well in the surgery, wanted me to be intubated for at least ten to twelve hours post-surgery, to make sure everything was functioning as it should and I wouldn't need the ventilator anymore. The last thing they wanted to do was to re-intubate me. But, having now tried to *stay calm* for nearing seven hours, and with things having shifted down in my throat due to the gagging, I wanted this large tube out *now*.

I began making motions with my hands, motions which still to this day I think were incredibly clear and accurate and which communicated what I wanted. In my head, I began making motions that mimicked the pulling of the tube out of my throat and mouth. But apparently, according to Kim and Lynette, my arms were pretty much just flailing around my head and face, and all it seemed I was doing was waving in a crazy manner. After a minute

Big Breath In

of questions, or trial and error about what I wanted, Lynette finally cracked my code: "You want your breathing tube out?" I nodded.

Thus began about twenty minutes of back-and-forth communication. My nurse saw and heard the exchange between Lynette and I, and came over herself to confirm what I was asking. She told me that even though I was doing a lot of the breathing on my own, it was still early to have the tube removed. She said she would call the doctor and see what he thought. A minute later, she came back and said that my doctors wanted to see me first and would be coming by soon to make an assessment.

Ten minutes passed and my nurse came back into view. My doctor had been called away and would not be able to come see me, but he saw that my numbers were good and that the respiratory therapist could go ahead and pull my tube. I looked over at Lynette, who was monitoring everything, wearing both her sister and nursing hats. I raised my eyebrows in an inquisitive fashion. She narrowed her eyes, looking at me in a calm, reassuring way and said, "You'll be okay." I gave her a quick nod, turned back to my nurse, and gave her the thumbs-up.

I don't remember the sensation or even the event of having my vent pulled, I think they increased my sedation drug before it, and I can't say it was an amazing feeling to have it out, as now my throat was very sore, but it was a nice sensation to not have that large tube down there, to be able to breathe on my own, and to be able to talk again, albeit in a raspy, barely audible whisper. The one thing I do remember is the thought that the surgery had been a success, and I was now breathing with the lungs of another person. Eight hours after surgery, at 2:00 p.m. on Saturday, June 19, I was off the ventilator and taking my first breaths with these new lungs all on my own.

I have no clear recollections of the following twenty hours. I have little pockets of memory. My parents came later that afternoon to see me. Kim's parents also saw me for a couple of minutes that afternoon. Kim was at my side all day. Lynette was in and out most of the day, and Bryan came to see me as well.

One thing that is clear in my memory is how much pain I was in and how uncomfortable I was. My back was sore and very itchy. I could only muster a whisper, I was sweating a lot, my hands and feet felt like they had pins and needles in them, and it was hard to breathe. Those first twenty-four hours were difficult, but they were also empowering. I had nothing to complain about, and the only thing I should have been feeling was immeasurable gratitude!

18.
RECOVERY: DAY 2

> "Less than two minutes later, when the sun emerged, the trailing edge of the shadow cone sped away.... it swept over the plain and dropped over the planet's rim in a twinkling. It had clobbered us, and now it roared away."
>
> (*Teaching a Stone to Talk,* Annie Dillard)

AFTER THE EXCITEMENT of getting off the ventilator and breathing on my own, I was left for the afternoon and evening to concentrate on the work set before me: *breathing on my own and staying off the ventilator!*

It sounds weird to say, but it was *work,* as I really did have to relearn how to breathe with these new lungs. Though they were in my body, they felt foreign, like they were not part of me yet. The only thing I can think to compare it to is like driving a brand-new car after only driving the same vehicle for twenty-years. You know what you're doing, but it no longer feels automatic, and you tend to overthink everything. However, though I was still in an incredible amount of pain and my chest was feeling very tight, like a belt was cinched around it, I felt that my oxygen capacity was much greater than the day before when I was waiting for surgery. There was also a new strength that I felt in my lungs. I felt as if I could pull oxygen deeper into my lungs with greater efficiency than the last couple years. It was not comfortable by any means because of the surgery I had undergone, but there was a new feeling of confidence in my chest. In the days to come, I would need to relearn how to cough, something I have heard many lung transplant patients struggle with. These lungs were new to me, and I had to figure out how to use them, to retrain my muscles to work with these new high-efficiency lungs.

Other than focusing on deep breathing, much of the rest of that first day is a blur. I was growing more and more uncomfortable in my bed. My back was itchy from all the sweating, and my feet were hurting because of nerve damage and swelling. But I was still quite sedated, which I was more than happy with.

Day two post-surgery consisted of a lot more work. When I woke up, or became conscious that it was daytime, my nurse mentioned they were going to get me up and out of bed, to try get me eating something. This was exciting news, as it meant things were progressing well.

By late morning, something new always seemed to be on the horizon. First, a physiotherapist came by at around 11:30 a.m. and said it was time to try to get me out of bed and sitting in a chair. By just lying in bed and resting from the surgery, my body was already starting to atrophy; therefore, movement was key, and since I was becoming more and more uncomfortable in bed, I was more than ready for this next step.

So far, the only thing removed since my surgery was my breathing tube, so I still had a plethora of lines coming out of me. The first step was to try to get me sitting on the edge of my bed, but of course with my chest having been popped open less than forty

Recovery: Day 2

hours earlier, I couldn't engage my muscles to sit up. First, the physio used the controls of my bed to get me in a sitting position. This took two people to do. One person, the physiotherapist, on my left side, pushing the button to raise the head of my bed while also keeping an eye that none of the lines coming out of me were getting caught or tugged or pulled anywhere, and a second person, my nurse, on the right side of me doing the same.

The second part of this complicated procedure was trying to swivel my body and get me to swing my legs off the left side of the bed. To do this, I kind of leaned over to my right and let my left leg drop off the side of the bed. The physio helped swivel my torso around, with my nurse guiding from behind, making sure all my lines were still loose. When I had turned almost 90 degrees, my physio carried my right leg down so that now both my legs were dangling off the side of the bed.

We were now about seven minutes into the procedure, and I was able to sit for a couple of minutes on the side of the bed to catch my breath and allow my blood to circulate around my body in this new position. I sat hunched over, with Kim holding my shoulder to ensure I didn't fall to the left or right, or sway too much forward or back.

A large chair was wheeled beside my bed. With my equilibrium returning and feeling more centered on the edge of the bed, it was now time to try standing. I suppose I should say, what happened next was not so much me standing as it was me being held in the arms of my physiotherapist as I tried to keep my legs under me, swiveling my hips so that my bare ass was pointed toward the chair that was waiting for me, and then allowing the physiotherapist to lower me back into a sitting position in the chair.

I don't remember much of the experience of standing, swiveling, and being lowered again. My mind focused on monitoring the growing pain I had and making sure no lines got caught up on anything. (You can tell by now, I was very concerned about all my lines.) But this simple procedure of standing and sitting again was work, and it might have been some of the most demanding work I had ever done in my life. I also knew it would have one of the biggest payoffs. If I could do this, I knew I would be on a trajectory that would lead to eating and drinking on my own, which would mean my NG tube coming out, which would mean I could then get out of the ICU and begin my journey of healing up on the ward, leading me eventually to getting back home and experiencing what this second chance at life held for me.

I sat in the chair for about fifteen minutes, and though it was somewhat painful, it also felt amazing to be out of the bed and off my back. During this whole time of sitting, Kim stood behind me with her hands placed on the front of my shoulders to ensure that I would not fall forward if I dozed off. My nurse changed my bed linens, which were soaked through with sweat and had pink and yellow dye all over them due to the disinfectant that had been spread all over my body during the surgery. After about fifteen minutes of sitting, my nurse suggested I try to eat something. With the feeding tube in, and with the general state I was in, it would still be days before I could try solid food, but I wanted to try this next step of recovery, as it would mean the nasty feeding tube could come out.

A small green plastic bowl of squash soup was placed in front of me. Kim grabbed a towel and tied it around my neck as a bib, as I am a messy eater, even at the best of times. As I looked at the soup, I got nervous, not because I worried about eating—like breathing on my own, I felt quite confident that I could do this—but I got nervous because I had never had squash soup before and I had always been a picky eater. I lifted the spoon to my mouth with a small puddle of soup in it, hand shaking like a paint mixer because of the high dose of steroids I was on. I sipped on the orange mush,

Recovery: Day 2

and I'll be damned if that wasn't one of the tastiest and most satisfying meals I have ever had. It wasn't so much that the VGH cafeteria makes the best squash soup (or maybe they do), but it had more to do with the fact that it had now been over two-and-a-half days since I had last eaten anything, and now here I was sitting up in a chair, only thirty hours after transplant, taking my first sips of food. That squash soup was a manifestation of where we had come from and the thrill, joy, and exhilaration I felt over the progress I was making. Even though I was still in a lot of pain, I could already see that my body wanted to begin the journey of healing, and maybe for the first time in years, it was finding within itself the strength and ability to do so.

I should mention, though, if I thought a lunch of squash soup was good, I was blown away at dinner: ice cream and yogurt! The reason for this dessert-dinner was that because the ventilator had now been removed, my throat was killing me, and the volume of my voice was down to that of a raspy whisper. To help numb and soothe the inside of my throat, I got these wonderful treats as my second meal. My nurse ended up having to take my yogurt away as I was eating more than I should; I couldn't hold back. For one of the first times in my life, I actually enjoyed eating.

Backing up a bit. After lunch, as I was sitting in the chair, squash soup now done, chin wiped clean, and I had proved I could eat and keep food in my stomach where it belonged, my nurse got the all-clear to remove my NG tube. This was maybe four of the most uncomfortable seconds in my life, as it rather feels like you are throwing up out of your nose. My nurse loosened the tape from the end of my nose, which held the tube in place. Then warning me to relax and breathe out, she began pulling, very much like you would, hand over hand, a long rope from out of a deep hole. As she came to the end, and the horror reached a crescendo with the tip of the tube moving up and tickling my gag reflex, she discarded the hand-over-hand technique and started pulling straight out into midair. We have a video of this happening, and even now, watching it over ten years later, it still makes me cringe.

By this time, I had been sitting for about forty-five minutes in the chair beside my ICU bed and my feet were getting quite sore as blood and fluid began pooling in them. They were really starting to swell up. I was transferred back into my bed, ever mindful of all my lines.

With all this fun now completed and seeing what my body was capable of, my doctor and the charge nurse of the ICU began talking about transferring me out of the ICU and up to the ward. This caught all of us a little by surprise, as I had only been in the ICU for a day and a half. The news brought excitement because this meant that my recovery was ahead of schedule, but also some fear and resistance, as I would be losing my one-on-one care. But as time progressed, I found myself more and more uncomfortable in my bed and found all my lines become more of a hassle. If a bed opened up on the thoracic ward, I would be moved.

With this now in the works, I began getting some of my lines removed, which I was quite happy about. The first thing out was one of my peripheral IV lines in my hand. Second was the arterial line in my wrist, which was always painful. Third was the femoral IV line in my groin. (I was not sad to see that one gone). Last, before moving up to the ward, the IVs in my neck were removed.

Around 7:30 p.m., just thirty hours after arriving in the ICU from surgery, word came down that a bed in a private room was ready for me. Again, I was happy that I had recovered to the point where the doctors and nurses felt comfortable with this move, but I had some anxiety about moving from a place where a set of nursing eyes were on me 24/7, to the ward where I would be in my

Recovery: Day 2

own room, under the care of a nurse who would have a couple of other patients to care for also.

In the end, I trusted my surgeon that it was time to take my next steps to recovery, to move out of my first residence with my new lungs, and to learn to be on my own and trust these new lungs and the nurses who would be caring for me. At around 7:30 p.m. on June 20, to much fanfare of all my sister's coworkers and even her boss, my bed was swung out of the ICU and down the long hallways to the elevators. I was brought back up to the twelfth floor, to the exact place I had come down from less than forty-eight hours earlier.

19.
RECOVERY STARTS AND STALLS

> "The essential thing 'in heaven and earth' is . . .
> that there should be a long obedience
> in the same direction;
> there thereby results, and has always
> resulted in the long run,
> something which has made life worth living."
>
> (*Beyond Good and Evil,* Friedrich Nietzsche)

I SPENT THE next two weeks, June 21 to July 5, in my own private room on the thoracic ward. My room was outstanding, especially compared to St. Paul's, as it had space for two beds. Because of my extreme immune suppression, they took the second bed out, so I had this very large room overlooking the beautiful downtown Vancouver skyline all to myself.

Like any recovery from major surgery, the big steps of recovery all happened within the first week. Each day marked a new milestone, with more lines being taken out of my body, and new forays into independence. But of course, after these giant leaps forward, the inevitable slowdown hit, progress plateaued, and the real work of recovery (two steps forward, one step back)—"a long obedience in the same direction"—really began.

One of my biggest struggles in moving up to the floor was getting used to the environment and the way they did things in this new (to me) hospital. I had spent so much time in St. Paul's (200 days and nights, to be exact) that I had become very familiar and friendly with all the nurses, doctors, lab techs, X-ray techs, and food service people. I knew how they operated, at what times things happened, and the level of care for the institution. And just as important, they also knew me. They knew what I could do, the level of independence I was capable of, and the level of anxiety I had about my care. They trusted me, and I trusted them.

But now, being in this different hospital, in this state of fragile health, everything was new. I was at the most vulnerable point I had ever been in my journey, not even being able to stand without the help of another person, and I had a hard time trusting what was going on around me with my care. I am the patient who is always double-checking nurses' work (which IV meds and pills are given), but I now felt totally out of control, as I was at the mercy of people I didn't know. I had to entrust myself to these people trusted to care for me.

Now, isn't this everyone's experience when admitted to hospital? Of course, but it hadn't felt like that for me at St. Paul's because it had become my home for the better part of the previous six months. So, needless to say, I very much drove my new nurse's crazy those first couple of days on the ward, always asking what they were doing and trying to double-check their work. My anxiety was running on overdrive.

Another thing that led to my anxiety was something I was not prepared for. I felt as if I was living in someone else's body. My body felt foreign to me for the first time in my life; in essence, I had to relearn what my body felt like and how to use it. It wasn't just that I still had four chest tubes, two IVs, a catheter, and was so drugged up on pain meds that I would fall asleep mid-sentence while talking to people, but the physical structure of my body also felt new.

There is an interesting phenomenon that people with CF often live with. We can often be very sick, our lungs at the point of failure, the line between being at home and needing to go into hospital razor thin, and yet we still have this ability to feel at home in our bodies and be comfortable living our lives. Our bodies, even while riddled with the end stages of CF and close to death, are still our home. They still move and function in ways we know and have adapted to for years, and we can still predict what they will do even when the state of our health is in a totally unpredictable situation.

However, after such an invasive and complex surgery, everything now felt different. Breathing, which should have been one of the most automatic things, all of a sudden became a conscious effort. I was feeling new sensations in my body. The effects of the surgery were numerous. My hands and feet were tingling with nerve pain and I had pain on the tops of my feet at the slightest touch of even the hair on them. It felt like two large leather straps were winched around my chest, and when I was laying down, it felt like a 45-pound bar was resting on my incision. I felt warm all the time, whereas I'd usually felt cold because of low oxygen saturation in my blood before my surgery. My voice was a raspy whisper, as my throat was parched and very painful. For the first forty-eight hours, each time I sat up, I would get the hiccups, which would rattle my whole body, sending shooting pain all over the place. Oh, and did I mention that no matter what they gave me, no matter how many suppositories I got, it would be over a week until I finally took a dump. That got uncomfortable real fast!

Big Breath In

That first week, and the following months, felt like I was relearning how to do everything. But the craziest part is that I would also go back to those first couple weeks in a heartbeat, it was such an exciting time!

Day 3, June 21, 2010: (Kim writing) *Quick update. George is doing awesome and better than expected. Lungs are doing well. He is fully conscious and questioning his nurses (as per usual). He isn't sleeping too well, but he is a trooper and continually improving.*

Day 5, June 23, 2010: (Kim writing) *George is still doing awesome! We are continually amazed at his quick progression. It has now been five days and he almost looks normal! Maybe even better than normal because he has more color. He has more mobility and appetite. Yesterday morning, he shuffled to the end of the hall and back. More and more tubes come out every day. He is now down to three chest tubes (he had four to begin with), a couple of IVs (one of which is his PICC line he has had for six months, so I'm not sure if it even counts!), and some supplemental oxygen. The pain is being managed pretty well so far. He is still very exhausted and can fall asleep when you're talking to him. No complaints or complications yet. The chest X-rays still look awesome. Thank you for your continued prayers and support once again!*

"Wait and See"

One of the biggest adjustments I had to make in those first days post-transplant was that not every setback with my lungs was cause for panic, or even needed to be addressed. My health situation was no longer critical. Before my surgery, when something seemed to be going sideways, the response was always to get on it

Recovery Starts and Stalls

right away before it spiraled out of control. Post-transplant, even in the acute recovery phase, I was beginning to hear the phrase, "Let's just wait and see." There was this new idea I needed to understand and accept, that my body now had the ability to heal itself in ways it hadn't had for years. It now had the oxygenated resources to fix minor problems on its own.

The first example of this was the morning after moving up to the floor, I felt a small air leak in my left lung. When I leaned forward or pushed on the lower-left part of my rib cage, my chest made a farting nose as air escaped through the incision of one of my chest tubes. My doctor said that this was normal, and they would "wait and see" how it went. Sure enough, after a week, it was gone.

One of the most uncomfortable experiences that greeted me each morning was my daily chest X-ray. Every morning at 4:30 a.m. (!!!), I would hear a large cart rolling down the hallways to my room. I didn't mind the early morning. I was usually already awake anyway due to the pain I was having. But the procedure of getting an X-ray was quite painful. I would first need to pull myself up from lying down using a rope tied to the end of my bed so that a large metal plate could be placed behind me. I would then let myself down to rest on the plate. The mobile X-ray machine would then be moved into position in front of me. I would then need some help from the technician to be adjusted and re-adjusted to make sure they could get a good shot. On a good morning, this would only take about five minutes. But on bad and painful mornings, it could take ten minutes or longer, depending on how good the X-ray tech was. From there, I would settle back into my snoozing sleep patterns until about 6:00 a.m., at which point I would turn on the TV and watch the news as a way to distract myself from the pain.

Day-to-Day-to-Day

Not a lot happened that first full day on the floor. It was a day to get settled in and adjusted to my new surroundings and the work that lay ahead of me. I vowed that first morning that for each meal, I would make myself get out of bed and sit in the large chair beside the bed, overlooking the Vancouver skyline. I still had my epidural and catheter in, so movement was somewhat complicated and executed very delicately, but my nurse helped me stand and pivot to the chair for those first couple of meals. My food was still in liquid form, but it was all very tasty. Within a day, due to the high dose of prednisone I was on, my appetite picked up and I found for the first time in my life that I loved eating. I had always said that if I could get all my nutrients by taking a pill, I would. Not anymore. In fact, like many transplant patients, I have come to have to watch my weight, as I love eating now. I rested for much of the day, slipping between sleeping and being awake. The day passed quickly, as my pain was managed well, and I was still exhausted.

That night, however, a new painful reality set in. I got about four hours of sleep in total, but my epidural stopped working at some point during the night. The order was to stop the epidural once it had run its course, so as the pain set in, I was given oral pain meds. However, with my high tolerance for most medication, it would take a while to get the pain fully under control and the right dosing titrated. Thus began a very uncomfortable number of days.

At 9:00 a.m. the following morning, day four of recovery (day two on the ward), the epidural was taken out. It was the right choice, and I soon came to appreciate not having it in, but I worried about how my pain would be managed. I knew pain was going to be part and parcel of my recovery, but that didn't make it any easier. I found, however, that I now had much more range in getting up and out of bed, being able to move around easier.

On that fourth morning, I also felt some rumblings in my lungs. It felt, and would be visibly confirmed in the coming days, that there was some pretty nasty mucus in these new lungs. However, as I mentioned before, I actually had to relearn how to cough as everything in my body felt new. At this point, that skill was still a day or two away as it would take some real effort and concentration to do this, something I had been doing non-stop for the last many years.

At around lunch that day, I had the first of my four chest tubes removed, which I took as a very positive sign. It meant that there was less fluid in my chest and that the lungs were heading in the right direction. After lunch, much to my relief, my catheter was also taken out. This made moving around much safer, in my mind.

The most exciting part of the day, however, came later in the afternoon when the physiotherapist came for a visit. She got me standing beside the bed and doing some shuffling around it, which felt great. She then surprised me by asking if I wanted to go for my first *real* walk. "Hell yeah," I said. "Let's take these new lungs for a spin!" Now the walk was only about fifty-feet, to the end of the nursing station and back, but to be on my feet, out of my room, and walking around without getting out of breath only four days out from surgery felt amazing! Yes, my feet hurt a lot due to nerve pain, something that would take a couple months to resolve, and my physiotherapist had to hold my arm as we walked along, but as I took these small shuffling steps, I saw it as another significant sign that this whole transplant thing might actually work out.

My fifth day post-surgery was huge, and it felt like I was on top of the world. At breakfast, I noticed that my appetite had come roaring back. I had been switched to an almost normal diet: back to my breakfast of oatmeal, eggs, and toast. I still had to be careful, making sure I chewed my food well, as parts of my throat were still quite numb from all the tubes that had been down there only a couple of days earlier, but it was good to be eating real food again.

My physiotherapist came by my room after breakfast, and together we walked around the whole twelfth floor! This was now the new measure of how far I could walk—how many laps of the whole floor (made up of two wards) I could do at a time or in a day. There were times during the day when the hallways seemed to turn into a bit of a race track with the number of patients doing laps around the floor, all of us pushing and pulling our IV poles with us. This first lap for me at 9:30 a.m., on June 23, 2010, would be the first of countless laps over the following days, and, of course, the first of many physical accomplishments I would set for myself in the years to come.

Due to this increased physical activity, the mucus in my lungs was starting to move, and by 11:00 a.m., I coughed up some of the nastiest stuff I had ever seen. It was a very strange thing to realize this phlegm I was now hacking up had most likely been in these lungs before I had received them. The phlegm was probably produced when the lungs began to fail, which made the surgeons almost call off the surgery. It was difficult to think of this back then, five days post-transplant. To tell you the truth, it is still difficult to think about now, the absolute complexity and intertwining of what happens in the midst of an organ transplant.

As the day continued, I was able to get my second chest tube removed. Both the chest tubes on my right side were now out, which at least meant I could try to sleep a little bit more on that side. My incision, which spanned my whole chest, from armpit to armpit, still sent shocks of pain throughout my body when I rolled over too far on my side, but it was nice to have some variety in sleeping. I rested for much of the afternoon, but at 4:30 p.m., Kim and I went for two more laps around floor.

This was a monumental day, and not only because of my appetite, the movement of mucus from my lungs, and all the walking, but the thing that made the day so memorable was that for the first time in almost a year, I was doing all this without the help of supplemental oxygen. After coming off the ventilator in the ICU, I was still on oxygen, but that fifth morning the oxygen prongs were taken off my nose before I went for my walk with the physio. We monitored my oxygen levels throughout the day, but as long as I took deep breaths, I was able to stay off the nose prongs. I was actually breathing without any help for the first time in over a year!

Unfortunately, as usually happens when one's body does something it is not accustomed to, I ended up paying the price for all that activity the following day. The pain in my chest amplified, and my feet started to feel like they were burning. I could only do one and a half laps around the floor that day (two steps forward, one step back).

My X-ray that morning also showed that I had some air caught between my right lung and the chest wall. It was a very weird sensation, as when I pressed on a certain area on the right side of my chest, it felt like there were Rice Krispies under my skin. The doctors assured me it was nothing to be concerned about. I once again had to trust that my body could now heal itself. Sure enough, after a of couple days, the snap, crackle, and pop disappeared.

Day 7, June 25, 2010: (Kim writing) *After all the changes in the first few days of recovery, it sort of feels like things are slowing down. After six days now, there is not much new to report. But that is also a good thing because it means there really isn't anything bad to report. No complications yet. Minor effects of the drugs but nothing*

Big Breath In

the doctors are worried about. He is getting a tiny bit more sleep at night. He is up and walking a few times a day and he is eating quite well. Managing the pain is his main focus at this time. But he is very positive and quite happy to just be sitting back in bed most of the day when he isn't being poked or prodded. Sitting back in bed is something he couldn't do without discomfort a week ago!

A week after transplant, my recovery slowed down and I began settling into some new rhythms. I was averaging about four to six laps around the floor each day, splitting them up in the morning and afternoon so as not to overdo it on my painful and swollen feet. The feeling in my chest was coming back; it was a feeling of numbness. To this day, there are small areas of my chest that are numb. As I was now moving around more, my body was getting used to these new sensations, and it felt like my lungs were trying to find their proper place in my chest. When I sat up, it was as if two metal plates were sliding over each other in my chest, one attached to my ribcage and the other attached to my abdomen, like you would imagine tectonic plates sliding past each other in an earthquake. At this time, I also began to hear, or more accurately *feel*, a clicking in my chest. When I would bring this and any other abnormal sensation up with my surgeon, he would remind me that all the X-rays and bloodwork looked good and that it had only been a week since I underwent major surgery. I needed to be patient and to let my body do its long work of recovery. I was now also down to only one chest tube and sleeping for about ninety minutes at a time, getting up to five hours of sleep in total, longer than I had ever slept in months.

Once we hit this one-week anniversary, the days also began to feel a lot longer. We started playing around with my pain meds, trying to find the right combination of long-acting meds but also taking breakthrough pain medication when needed. I was now moving around a lot, maybe doing more than I should have. All the new movements I was engaging in were leading to more pain, especially around the incision, which then led me to take more pain meds. Subsequently, some of these days around the one-week mark I spent snowed under from the pain meds. I would get up and walk a couple of laps around the floor, get back to my room, lie down, and within moments I would be asleep, or at least in that gross state of being half-awake and half-asleep. It would take a good four days before we found the right balance of being comfortable but not always groggy.

On the Saturday morning (eight days post-surgery), my final chest tube was clamped. Later in the afternoon, my surgeon came by and looked at the clamped tube. He removed the clamp, and sure enough, some fluid and air came out, so he decided to keep it open for at least one more night.

The following day, June 27, it was apparent that very little fluid and air were escaping through this last tube, and anything left could be absorbed by my body. My nurse pulled the last chest tube. Freedom at last!

The next night, Monday night, I put my newfound freedom to use and did something I had not done before. With the last chest tube out, I was no longer attached to anything. I was not on antibiotics anymore, no catheter, no heart-rate monitor. So, as Kim was leaving to go home that night, I actually (drumroll, please) walked her to the elevator! Impressed? Yeah, probably not. But for me, it was something to celebrate. By now, I was doing multiple laps around the floor at one time, so it wasn't so much the distance that was impressive—far from it—but it was the fact that I could now do it. Before this, anytime I got off my bed, it was always a bit of a chore with all my lines and IV pole. But as Kim was packing up and getting ready to leave, as she kissed me goodnight and began walking to the door, I simply stood up out of bed, slid my swollen feet into my sandals, and started walking. No oxygen needed to be changed over to the portable tank, no IV pole to unplug and haul around, no chest tubes hanging below my gown, or heart-rate monitor to grab and pin up—I just got up and strolled along beside her.

It sounds stupid, but this was one of the most significant milestones of my recovery. And I can still remember the feeling of exhilaration I had walking back to my room, that this was now so easy to do. I was no longer trapped, no longer a prisoner to my body, my bed, or to the lines coming out of my body. I was recovering from a double-lung transplant, and at least for this night, everything was all right.

The following day, however, came with my first setback. As mentioned before, I would begin each day with a 4:30 a.m. chest X-ray. The main reason for this was to make sure no inflammation was developing. Acute rejection, which is most likely to occur in the first couple of months post-transplant, is the development of rapid inflammation in the lungs. When my doctor came to visit me later in the morning, she said that the X-ray from earlier that morning showed that there might be the development of some inflammation. This was not a big deal. Some inflammation is always normal, but she decided to take a preventative measure and upped my dose of steroids to try to keep it in check. The next morning, however, when my X-ray was checked, it looked like the inflammation was already down, as the picture of my lungs was not as fuzzy as it had looked the day before.

It was now Wednesday, twelve days post-transplant. I decided it was time to set some goals for myself. I began upping my number of laps around the floor and trying to add some speed. I did four laps in ten minutes in the morning, repeating this feat in the afternoon. That evening, I not only walked Kim to the elevators, but I walked her all the way to the front doors of the hospital. I was hooked up to my IV pole that evening, getting some needed fluids, but I decided, with the permission of my nurse, that I wanted to finally get off the floor. I masked and gloved up before taking the elevator down to the main lobby. We walked around the lobby for a couple of minutes, ducked outside so I could take in my first gulps of fresh air with my new lungs, smell the lovely exhaust fumes of all the cars driving past the hospital, and then, for fun, walked to the bottom of a ramp so I could see how I would do on an incline. I got up the ramp, but it was clear that my legs still had a long way to go in their recovery.

However, these goals of distance, ramps, and speed all paled compared to the goal my doctor set for me, which was to try to be discharged from hospital less than a week from that day. This meant I'd be going home less than three weeks after my transplant.

The following five days came with a lot of pain, both physical and mental. But with my sights now set on discharge, it was all I could think about. We were now looking forward to going home, but we also knew I was not yet ready to cross that bridge. We still had to be patient. Add to this that we were entering a long weekend, and life in the hospital was slowing right down.

Day thirteen of my recovery, July 1, was very slow. This is Canada Day, and like most any other business, a hospital slows down considerably on the big holidays. We were still trying to get my pain under control with the long- and short-acting pills. Due to my pain level, I decided to take the day off from walking around the floor, resting my still-swollen legs.

The titrating of pain meds continued for another two days. I would wake up in pain in the morning, take medication to try to bring the pain level down, take one too many pills, find myself a

Big Breath In

walking zombie for most of the day, then experiencing pain again once the meds wore off. Then, not wanting to repeat this zombie state, I would not take enough pain meds when the pain came on, and so I'd be in too much pain the following day. By this time, the pain would be so bad I wouldn't want to move or get up and walk. I'd try to catch up on my pain meds and again take too many, and then once again slip back into my zombie state. To help with some of this, instead of taking pain meds at night, I was instead switched to sleeping pills, which ended up doing the trick to balance things out. This was the first time I had ever taken a sleeping pill, as I had always heard they could be addicting, but I had finally had enough with the bad sleeps and snowed-under days. It ended up working quite well. I was able to rest better when I needed, take fewer pain meds, and over the course of the weekend, things began to even out.

Because I was getting more active, the biggest source of discomfort other than my incision was my feet. I would try to elevate them while in bed and try walking in place or massaging them throughout the day, but it wasn't until I went home and was more up and about that the swelling finally started going down.

The highlight of these last couple of days in hospital was Lynette's return to work. Now that I was on the road to recovery and soon to be heading home, she decided to return to work, as she had already been cleared to do so once I left the ICU. About a year before my transplant, she had a slight change in her job description, and instead of being at the bedside of an ICU patient all the time, she instead had a role on the critical care outreach team. This meant she would respond to calls from anywhere in the hospital when a patient was potentially crashing and where the patient's nurse thought the person might need to be moved to the ICU. Lynette, along with a respiratory therapist, would respond to any call from any floor to assess the patient, and then make the call if the patient should be transferred down to the ICU or if they could stay where they were for the time being. She would also check on patients who had recently been sent up from the ICU to their respective floors to make sure they were still recovering well.

Therefore, when Lynette returned to work, I was able to see her throughout the day as she checked on patients on the floor I was on. She would also poke her head into my room to see if I was awake both before and after her shift. At that time, I made a note in my journal. *Even though Lynette has been nursing for over 10 years, I have never seen her in action. It was fun to see her in her element. I don't think there was a prouder patient in the hospital.*

As Sunday night turned into Monday morning, I woke up with a spirit of anticipation. Having been in the hospital over the long weekend, I now felt that I had been in a day or two longer than I needed to be and I wanted out. I had learned a week earlier how to take all my anti-rejection meds on my own. All my lines, other than my PICC line, which I'd had since January, had been removed. I was steady on my feet. I was still in some pain but was managing well with the meds I was on. I could shower, change, eat, piss, and poop all on my own. (Yes, imagine a proud, wide-smiling toddler.) Everything was working and moving, and now it was time to begin the next stage of my health journey: out-patient recovery!

It was July 5, and I had now been in hospital since May 17. Thankfully, I was not the only one who felt it was time for me to go home. Right away in the morning, the wheels began turning to get me discharged. After breakfast, I was sent down for an X-ray. No longer did the portable X-ray machine come to my room at 4:30 a.m., but it had been decided a couple of days earlier that I had probably had enough X-rays to last me a lifetime. We could begin

Big Breath In

reducing the number I was receiving and I would go downstairs for them.

In the later morning, we began doing some of the baseline testing that I would get done each year following my transplant. We did the six-minute walking test, which is exactly what it sounds like—I would walk for six minutes and see how far I could get, having my heart rate, blood pressure, and oxygen saturation monitored while doing it.

The day ended up stretching on quite long. There was confusion with what blood work needed to be done before going home. I ended up having blood drawn three times that afternoon. There was confusion about what meds could be stopped and what meds I needed to take home with me. I also had not seen the doctor yet, so as the hours ticked by, we began getting more and more anxious and frustrated that this discharge might not happen. However, at the eleventh hour, which was around 4:30 p.m., my doctor finally appeared. He was almost as surprised to see me sitting on the edge of my bed as I was to see him in my room so late in the day. With a chuckle and confused look on his face, he asked what I was still doing there. He had just got back from a long weekend holiday and thought that one of the other doctors had taken care of getting me out. Alas, that communication was never received. With the lightning speed that only a veteran doctor could command, brown bags full of transplant medications were rushed up from the pharmacy, paperwork was filled out, and Kim and I were briefed on a binder filled with pages of instructions and phone numbers. I was then given an appointment card for the following morning, to be at the post-transplant clinic across the street from the hospital at 7:30 a.m.

Those last thirty minutes of hospitalization were pure pandemonium. My anxiety about leaving the hospital hit an all-time high as I was having a hard time keeping everything straight in my head. I can only imagine that what I was feeling was similar to first-time parents bringing their newborn baby home—was I really allowed the leave the hospital with this delicate and fragile new thing? Was my professional nursing care actually over? Was it just Kim and I and my new lungs now? But as the doctor left the room and the last nurse said her goodbye and walked out of my hospital room, Kim and I just looked at each other, smiled, and said, "Okay, I guess we can go home then."

To say that this moment was surreal would probably be the understatement of my life. I slipped off my hospital slippers for the last time and put on the old athletic sandals that Kim had brought in. I watched Kim pick up my duffle bag and knapsack. She then turned and looked at me as I stood up from the chair. We both smiled with raised eyebrows, glanced over to the door, and just started walking. Leaving the long history of hospital rooms behind us was exhilarating!

It was a warm afternoon as we walked out the hospital doors. The sun was shining, with only a few clouds in the sky. I was wearing my old blue jeans, which were now a couple of sizes too big because of all the weight I had lost, and my navy-blue Seattle Seahawks T-shirt. We came to the place on the landing right before it rises over the street. I looked back at Kim, who was following a few steps behind me. This was the place I had always stopped when I would walk Kim out in the evening. This was the edge of the hospital property. After this, I was in a public city space.

I fixed my eyes forward, took a step over that invisible line, and then another. The prison of my failing health, my doomed lungs that had kept me bound and shackled for the previous four years, the waiting for transplant for over eighteen and a half months, the seventeen days of hospital recovery—all of that was now over. It was time to walk headlong into the new life that awaited me. I knew I still had a long way to go. It would be another seven months before I would feel like myself again, and it would be almost a year before I would begin living what could pass for a "normal" life of someone my age.

But as I took that first step off the hospital grounds, I knew I was walking into a new opportunity, a new adventure, a new life with new dreams and new possibilities. I could begin to think and dream of a future that I'd never thought possible just a couple of weeks earlier. Only seventeen days prior, an ambulance had dropped me off on the other side of the hospital, taking me through the emergency department on my way to get my transplant. We didn't know if that would be the last day of my life or first day of a new one. And now, seventeen days into this new life, this second chance at life, we were moving forward again, into the unknown.

I began walking over the pedestrian overpass. Halfway over, I looked back. Kim had the camera out and was filming me, walking and smiling, walking and laughing. I was out! I had been given a second chance. I had received the precious *gift of life*.

20.
EPILOGUE

"The only real difference between people is not health or illness but the way each holds onto a sense of value in life. When I feel I have no time to walk out and watch the sunlight on the river, my recovery has gone too far. A little fear is all right. It is all right to know that in a month I could be lying in a hospital bed asking myself how I spent today... When the ordinary becomes frustrating, I have to remember those times when the ordinary was forbidden to me. When I was ill, all I wanted was to get back into the ordinary flux of activity. Now that I am back in the ordinary, I have to retain a sense of wonder at being here."

(*At the Will of the Body*, Arthur W. Frank)

JULY 6, 2010: *Well day one at home is done, and it was a surprisingly relaxing day. I had my first Transplant Clinic visit today and will be going to clinic twice a week for the next couple months. Yesterday, when being discharged, the transplant doctor warned us that today at clinic was going to be crazy, but it actually went quite* well. We were out of there in four hours, which sounds like a while but was actually very fast.

The best experience was meeting other lung transplant recipients. There is a woman who had a double-lung transplant two weeks before me, and another man who had a single just hours after me. The woman was discharged at the end of last week and the man was discharged yesterday, the same as me. So, for all three of us it was our first clinic, so it was really fun to talk for a bit and share some stories. It was really good to wander through this new experience with some other "rookies." In order to get all the tests done we have to navigate four different floors of the Diamond Center at VGH, so it was a little confusing, but we should have a better handle on it next time.

It is now about 8:30 p.m., and Kim and I just got in from a 20-minute sunset walk on the dyke, something we haven't done since we started dating and even then it was hard for me, so being able to eat a big dinner and go out for a walk is so amazing it almost brings tears to my eyes.

July 10, 2010: We are continually amazed at how things are going and how life is when I am not having to constantly do physio. All of a sudden I have an extra six hours in my day that used to be filled with physio. Kim and I actually started watching a movie at 8:00 p.m. last night for the first time in . . . ever probably, because I didn't have to go and do physio from 8:00 to 9:30.

July 19, 2010: Well yesterday marked one month since my transplant and I still can't believe the difference from last month to this month. We had a great weekend at home. We had some family over, some friends over and we even went for a walk in Watershed Park. It was quite amazing to be hiking and out of breath but still able to keep walking like an ordinary person. The whole time we were *walking, I just couldn't help but be in disbelief that I could be doing this. Of course, after the 30-minute walk, with a bunch of rests, I was totally done for the day but it was amazing to experience that.*

August 5, 2010: *I am not having much pain from my incision anymore. I am still on some pain meds though, but it is more for my foot and hand. My right foot and left hand both seem to have some nerve damage from the surgery. It is nothing new and the doctors have seen it before. But it is a bit uncomfortable. It was really starting to get aggravated when I was walking more, but now I have started biking and that seems to help.*

October 7, 2010: *Things have been going very well. Kim and I have taken up biking a little bit and on weekends when the weather is nice, we have also done a lot of walking. The Lower Mainland has so many beautiful places to explore; it truly is an amazing place to live with so many beautiful places within an hour's driving distance. It has been three weeks since I have been to the transplant clinic, so that is a good sign. My mind is back to a place where I can start reading again without falling asleep, and for the first time in my life, I enjoy reading more than watching TV. I am feeling more and more comfortable in what feels like a whole new body, not just new lungs. My incision is slowly starting to heal over in some places and I think by the end it should not be very noticeable at all, at least that is the goal.*

October 18, 2010: *I just got off the treadmill after what has become a pretty routine afternoon workout of cardio and strength training. For the past three or four years, or maybe even longer, I have had a deep fear and hatred of stairs and any sort of incline. So, during my workouts now, I am concentrating on strength training and when I am on the treadmill I always make sure there is an ever-increasing*

incline. *I feel the need to overcompensate for my previous fear of stairs and hills by never becoming embarrassed by them again!!*
It is amazing how things have changed over the past four months. I feel a new freedom that I have not felt in years. Coming from a dairy farm, I will use this analogy. I feel like a heifer-calf entering a large new pen for the first time. I will go bounding, leaping and jumping into it, then stop suddenly, look around, take a tentative step or two, take another jump or two, stop again, sniff around tentatively, walk a couple more steps, stand still for a while not moving no matter how much I am encouraged, and then slowly settle down, becoming more comfortable with my new surroundings.

It has been a journey in which I struggle to find the words to adequately describe it, each time feeling that I am not doing it justice with my limited vocabulary. Last night we had some friends over to watch the game, and after they left, I sat down behind the computer, opened up our iTunes library, and put some music on. Before getting back up to help with the dishes, Kim said, "You going to do physio then?" It was a joke we both laughed at, but a reminder of how many hundreds of times I have sat there doing my physio. It is amazing how much our lives have changed, how our life was before transplant, and how it is now.

December 17, 2010: *I wanted to write today and give an update (for those of you still reading along), as tomorrow will mark six months post-transplant.*
Things have been going well for the most part over the last two months. Throughout the end of October and first half of November, I was dealing with a lot of chest pain, which was discouraging. It was due to the muscles in my chest getting back into shape, or should I say, back to basic use. I kept pulling my chest muscles over and over again with just normal things. I haven't done any normal lifting in such a long time that it was quite the shock to my body when I

did. I have to be patient. The pain has gone away for the most part, as now I am doing a lot of stretching and being more careful when lifting anything.

Kim and I are really enjoying this Christmas season. Last year, I spent Christmas in St. Paul's hospital. Granted I did get a pass for actual Christmas Day, but all the lead-up to Christmas was spent in the hospital. Surprisingly, my memories of that time are not all bad. Obviously, it was not fun, but we made the most of it. God gave us the attitude to get through that time. Of course, it doesn't compare to this year. Life now seems so free. Being able to go here and there. Being able to help Kim with all the Christmas happenings. Decorating the house, doing some shopping, and we even put lights on the outside of our house for the first time. I have also started doing a bit of cooking, which is totally new for me. But it is kind of fun, and it doesn't taste too bad either! Again, we are so thankful. We again want to thank all of you for your thoughts, encouragement, and prayers. We want to thank the transplant team that has done so much for us over the past six months. Also, for the care and expertise of the CF team at St. Paul's, for all that they did to keep me going during the first half of this year and all of last year.

It has been an amazing year. Many ups and downs, very emotional and very exciting. We continue to take it day by day, as we still become more and more comfortable with post-transplant living.

My View Today (Spring 2021)

The years following my transplant were years of exciting new experiences. Being immunocompromised, once I learned how to safely push the boundaries of what I was comfortable with, life opened up into opportunities I never thought possible.

Big Breath In

Ten months after my transplant, I enrolled in graduate school to begin working on a master's degree. I studied part time while also working, taking five years to finish the 90-credit program, opening the way for me to become an ordained pastor.

On my one-year transplant anniversary (*transplantiversary*), Kim's brother, Paul, and I hiked the Grouse Grind, a hike up one of Vancouver's local mountains. It is only a 2.9-kilometer hike, but it gains 853 meters of elevation while ascending 2,830 steps up the side of the mountain.

Soon after this, I got into road cycling. At the end of 2011, I began a year and a half of training in order to participate in a CF fundraiser called GearUp4CF. This fundraiser was a nine-day, 1,200-kilometer ride from Vancouver, BC, to Banff, Alberta. I completed the ride in 2013 and again in 2014, each time riding with about twenty-one other riders. After this, I got into mountain biking, riding about three times a week, until a serious crash in 2019, where I found myself having to walk out of the forest clutching my limp right arm with a bone sticking out of it, caused me to reevaluate some of my more *overachieving* hobbies.

I have had opportunities to engage in many public speaking roles, sharing about CF, transplant, and person-centered-care, from small networking lunches to university classrooms to international health-care conferences.

Kim and I have gone camping each summer and have been lucky enough to travel to sun-filled destinations most winters. Post-transplant living has been like nothing I could have ever imagined.

But life is complex, and though it can be filled with the most incredible beauty and joy, it can also be filled with heartache, sorrow, and suffering. As I write these words, now, some eleven years since my transplant, life has once again been filled with medical appointments, hospital beds, and more medications than I can sometimes keep track of. But this time, the medications and appointments aren't for me; they have been for Kim. My transplant has given me some incredible roles and opportunities in life, but none more so than the honor of being a caregiver for my wife, who passed away on April 2, 2021, after a five-year journey with cancer.

I admit that there are times when my life story seems too much. Warren—CF—transplant—cancer. In my more depressive moments, it sometimes seems like I am just moving from one loss to another, that everything I touch is taken away. The resiliency that was part and parcel of our home growing up, which I learned and witnessed in Warren and sought to put into practice after his death, seems to be running low these days as I have watched the love of my life, my constant companion, the one who got me through my darkest days, now taken from me. The weight of sorrow that I first saw in my parents' eyes after Warren passed away, I now see in my own eyes when I look in the mirror.

And yet, Warren's legacy of strength and courage, gratitude and determination in the face of adversity, even in the face of the terminal, I know still resides somewhere within. It is just more silent and hidden these days. For as my dad said recently, with tears running down his cheeks, "We have been through so much already, but we will not let this beat us."

A constant theme I have found myself having to grapple with for most of my adult life, and which is written between the lines of this book, is having to continually learn to live in the unknown. I have spent so much time standing on what feels like quicksand that I have often longed to just stand on some consistently solid ground, some sort of "ordinary" kind of life. But I have had to accept that much of my life has been about adapting to and accepting the unknown, learning to live in the ever-changing circumstances that life keeps bringing my way, and now learning to do that by myself. And the struggle in this, as Arthur Frank writes, whom I quoted to begin this chapter, is trying to hold on to a "sense of value" in these disorientating times.

There will come a time, or many times, or even a cruel number of times, when you will need to face your own seasons of unknowingness, and maybe accept for yourselves a reality you don't want to. There are things in life that we don't get a choice in. But how we face those unknowns, whether we will run in fear and keep our head down in denial, or whether we will grieve what has been lost (often for a significant amount of time) and then face those unknowns head-on, seeking to find new value and meaning, is ultimately up to us.

There have been times, recently, watching Kim suffer and now with her gone, when I hate the life I have been given. I wonder, with a pain-filled heart, what it would be like to have lived a "normal" life—to not have known the death of my brother, to not have known of CF and the horrors it can inflict on the body, to not have known what it is like to wait for an organ transplant, and to not have known the gut-wrenching work of caregiving for a most-loved-one with cancer, sitting with her until the very end, watching and listening to her exhale her very last breath. But I try not to stay in that place too long because there has also been blessing and even gratitude in the ever-changing story I have been given. I miss Kim so much, but I am also so thankful for every moment we had together, even the difficult ones.

My story of CF and transplantation has been one of constant change and a persistent need to navigate a foggy horizon. Sometimes I have done this well, keeping my sense of value and meaning even when it seemed life was passing me by, but mostly, it has been a very difficult road to travel. Overall though, I am grateful for experiences of CF and transplantation, and the sense of value, dedication, and strength they have given me. It was, after all, those experiences that gave me the ability and strength to walk

Epilogue

with and care for Kim these last years—and to now try continue on without her.

As I mentioned in the first pages of this book, we as humans love stories. They can help us put the pieces of our life together. I hope that my story of ups and downs, of facing the unknowns of living with CF, and the unique experience of receiving a double-lung transplant has in some way been able to serve you. I hope it has been a companion for you, a support in your own journey—or maybe it has just provided a couple of hours of distraction and a few laughs, destined for the second-hand bookstore; that's okay, too. Whatever it has meant, I hope that in some way it will help strengthen your story of past and present and that it might aid you in facing the future—even a very unknown one.

ACKNOWLEDGEMENTS

IT IS IMPOSSIBLE to try and name the hundreds of people who have contributed to this story, whose encouragement, phone calls, text messages, emails and prayers have helped guide me through my life. It has truly taken a village to bring me to the place I am today. However, I will try name a few people who have tangibly helped bring this book to fruition.

First off, I owe a debt of gratitude to the team at FriesenPress. To my publishing team and editors, thank you for all your patience, extended deadlines, professionalism, and feedback. Hannah, thank you for bringing me into the FriesenPress family. Since speaking with you at the very beginning of this process, I have never doubted my choice of publisher.

Thank you to all those over the years who have encouraged me to write and to all those at Providence Health Care in Vancouver who have heard me speak or read my articles and reached out to tell me to get my story down on paper.

To my recent conversation partners, Leanne Stam, Margot Vegt, Margaret Hummelman, and Sophie Nagtegaal, your encouragement in the months leading up to the COVID-19 pandemic to write was paramount to finally getting this project underway.

Big Breath In

Thank you to the congregation of Bridge Community Church in Langley, BC, for giving me the time and space to write once the pandemic hit. Thank you for your patience in listening to my sermons every Sunday morning for three years, where I learned how to hone my writing and storytelling ability (as deficient as it still is).

Thank you, Glenda Konrad, for being my first unofficial editor and whose feedback gave me the confidence to forge ahead. Your early advice and encouragement meant everything to me. To Sonja Rietkerk, it was your palpable interest in this project that finally made me realize that it could one day be published. To Heidi Rietkerk, your enthusiasm and willingness to provide insightful feedback, from cover design to reading the manuscript and providing critical comment, came at a time when I had lost all confidence in myself and felt very alone. Thank you for your willingness to help and your enthusiasm along the way!

To all my in-laws—Brian and Florence Rietkerk, Paul and Sonja, Tim and Heidi—thank you for your unconditional acceptance and love; for all your support in my thirteen years with Kim and your steadfastness in the months since she has been gone.

To my amazing family: My parents, Art and Wilma Keulen, thank you for loving me, understanding me, and walking with me in all things. You have given me nothing but good things in this life, and I am so thankful that you are my parents. To Lynette, you have endured so much in walking beside me, protecting and caring for me from a young age. I could never have asked for a better sister. And to Bryan, you have been a pillar of strength and commitment since the moment you joined the family. You are not only strong in physique but even more so in heart and spirit.

To Eliza, Charlotte, Jack, Lauren, Matthew, Julia, Harrison and Jackson, you have all brought so much joy to your Uncle George and Aunty Kim. We love you so much!

Acknowledgements

I owe the endurance of my CF lungs to the CF Team at St. Paul's Hospital in Vancouver. You saw me through my darkest days, never giving up on me, and always making sure I had the best care possible. A special thanks to Brigette and Pat, your compassion not only kept my lungs going, but my spirit as well.

And I owe the functioning of my transplant lungs to the team at BC Transplant. From the first meet-and-greet to my latest clinic visit, you are keeping these lungs inside of me going. Your expertise and dedication to the field of lung transplants has helped so many lives flourish into something many of us never thought possible.

There are no words that can come close to appropriately thanking my donor and donor family. Every breath I have taken since receiving the precious gift of these lungs is owed to you! It is my hope that I have lived my life these past eleven years in a way that is honoring to you and worthy of the life that was lost on that fateful day.

And lastly, to Kim, I would never have seen my transplant day if it wasn't for you—your love, your commitment, your service, your support. We went through so much those first years of marriage, and yet you never complained, your love never faltered, and you never made me feel inadequate. You were always there. I have tried my hardest these past years to be for you what you were for me, but I know I came up short so many times compared with what you did for me. As we always said, you made the better caregiver, I made the better patient. Every page of this book is for you. You read through all the early drafts and made me keep writing because you wanted to read more. This book would never have happened without you. On the day you were diagnosed for the last time, driving home from the cancer clinic, you made me promise to finish this book. The only reason it is done today is because of that promise. It is all for you. I still don't know how I will continue on without you. I love you, and I miss you so much. *I'll see you in a bit.*

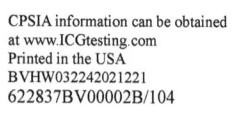

CPSIA information can be obtained
at www.ICGtesting.com
Printed in the USA
BVHW032242021221
622837BV00002B/104

9 781039 111462